I0803035

Who's Your Doctor?

A Guide to Protect You From the Wrong One

WILLIAM ABRAMOVITS, MD, FAAD

SAVIO REPVBLIC

A SAVIO REPUBLIC BOOK
An Imprint of Post Hill Press
ISBN: 979-8-89565-047-9
ISBN (eBook): 979-8-89565-048-6

Cover Design by Jim Villaflores
Asclepius attribution: Vecteezy.com

This book contains advice and information relating to health care. It should be used to supplement rather than replace the advice of your doctor or another trained health professional. You are advised to consult your health professional with regard to matters related to your health, and in particular regarding matters that may require diagnosis or medical attention. All efforts have been made to assure the accuracy of the information in this book as of the date of publication. The publisher and the author disclaim liability for any medical outcomes that may occur as a result of applying the methods suggested in this book.

This is a work of nonfiction. All people, locations, events, and situations are portrayed to the best of the author's memory.

SAVIO REPVBLIC Post Hill PRESS

posthillpress.com
New York • Nashville
Published in the United States of America

1 2 3 4 5 6 7 8 9 10

Contents

Advance Praise for *Who's Your Doctor?*

"In the past, when a person sought medical, not 'health' care, they either visited or were visited during a house call by a doctor who was often assisted by a nurse. There was no health insurance, and the doctor charged a fee for the provided service. Sometimes, that fee was paid not just in cash but also in goods, including food.

"Today, 'medicine' is seldom referred to as a profession, and physicians are called 'healthcare providers.' Doctors are no longer the primary caregivers for many patients treated solely by physician assistants or nurse practitioners. Some individuals in the 'healthcare industry' lack medical training but make decisions that impact millions of lives every day. Social media 'influencers' promote health concepts, treatments, and products without scientific evidence to support their efficacy or safety. Billions are spent on television ads for medications. At the same time, other companies offer online prescriptions through virtual providers who make them available with little, if any, interaction with a doctor, often resulting in unexpected and harmful side effects. Third-party payers now dictate doctors' earnings, often reimbursing below the costs necessary to provide care.

"These factors have created a chaotic system that is more complex than in previous years. Patients and their families often find themselves confused and unsure about navigating a dizzying and daunting morass. In this book, my good friend and colleague, Dr. William Abramovits, has authored a pithy yet clear text that can assist patients in their interactions with the healthcare system. As evident from the first few pages, William is 'old school' and was trained classically before the advent of the internet, managed care, and large insurance conglomerates. He believes that physicians should be the primary providers of medical care, and he sees each of his patients, a practice he has maintained for many decades.

"Readers will value candid and honest discussions on various important topics and emerge better educated and equipped to 'do battle' with what has transformed from a simple doctor-patient interaction into a monstrous hydra."

—Clay J.Cockerell, MD, FAAD, MBA, JD., Chair, Department of Dermatology, Lake Granbury Residency Program, Past-President and Secretary-Treasurer, American Academy of Dermatology

"Bill can never be accused of mincing words. In *Who's Your Doctor?*, he takes on the pseudo-doctors and pseudo-treatments with which our patients are inundated, beginning with the premise: 'Readers will have to believe me over the crooks intent on taking money from sick and desperate people in need of medical care.' Dr. Abramovits's style is witty and engaging as he takes on complementary and alternative medicine (CAM) doctors and naturopathic physicians, among others. His summary of their activities is glib, to the point, and undoubtedly true: 'What these characters provide are alternatives to evidence-based, best available proven medicine.'

"Bill takes on clinics offering 'quasi-miracles,' like shots for weight loss, treatments that guarantee youth, make hair grow, or substitute for knee replacement surgery. He made me recall a Letterman monologue in which he poked fun at an ad for weight loss without diet or exercise; according to David, the only other option was disease! I was also reminded of a sign in a rice pudding store in Manhattan: 'If you want to look young and thin, hang out with old fat people!'

"Dr. Abramovits laments the proliferation of clinics in Walgreens, CVS, and other pharmacies where nurse practitioners (NP) or physician assistants (PA) distribute medical advice and opinions, often unsupervised and without the rigorous medical training of MDs and DOs. He points out that the Affordable Care Act shields such 'mid-levels' from malpractice suits because a doctor-patient relationship is not established at such locations.

"Dr. Abramovits is particularly harsh on CAM, pointing out that 1.5 percent of total health expenditures in the US are wasted on it; in 2007, that was almost $40 billion. He doesn't spare homeopathy, chelation, and Reiki, lumped with voodoo, colonics, and snake oil. On homeopathic remedies, he is blunt: 'They contain almost nothing therapeutic, which explains why they are safe and about as effective as placebo.' Chelation is referred to as unethical, dangerous, and, again, no better than a placebo; his caution is straightforward: 'Steer away from chelation therapy, unless prescribed by a medical doctor for its approved indication, namely metal poisoning.' Acupuncture gets off a bit easier, 'a questionable last resort for pain not alleviated with conventional therapies' that should only be practiced by 'competent and experienced anesthesiologists.' In unrelenting but completely factual and humorous style, Bill takes on reflexology: 'If you are not charged more than for a foot massage, enjoy, just don't count on it to be a cure for anything.' I particularly enjoyed his comments about cupping, which reminded me of a Yiddish saying I heard as a child to describe a useless activity: *Se velt helfen vie a toiten bankes*, roughly translating into 'It's about as effective as cupping is for a dead person.' If the issues weren't so sad, this would make for great comedy; I'm waiting for Dr. Abramovits to sign with *Saturday Night Live*!

"On a serious note, Dr. Abramovits discusses the training requirements for different health-care providers, including physicians, NPs, PAs, chiropractors, osteopaths, and so on. He gives fair appraisals of podiatrists, anesthetists, and midwives; naturopaths don't fare well; nutritionists come out okay. Although Bill expresses real concerns about NPs and PAs posing as physicians, he does not question that they can significantly help doctors.

"He warns readers to be leery of the American Board of Physicians Specialties (ABPS), which I've always viewed as the board that certifies individuals who couldn't pass the board exams sanctioned by the American Board of Medical Specialties (ABMS). As he points out, some states don't allow individuals only certified by the ABPS to advertise they are board-certified.

"Bill tackles turf collusions between optometrists and ophthalmologists, podiatrists and orthopedic surgeons, chiropractors and physiatrists, and psychologists and psychiatrists.

"The book has a tremendous common-sense section on how to find a doctor: Your doctor should be board-certified, recommendations should be sought, and you should go to specialists when you know which one is needed to get an expert on a condition. If you need to know what specialist you need, family practitioners, internists, gynecologists, and pediatricians can help. You should also check the doctor's status with his state medical board and more.

"The book is written for the lay public and explains much information that most non-medical consumers need to know about the health-care system. Even as a physician, I learned a lot. Equally important, Dr. Abramovits' humor and wit kept me entertained."

—Mark Lebwohl, MD, FAAD, President,
American Academy of Dermatology, Chair, New
York Mt. Sinai Hospital Dermatology Department

"My lifelong friend William Abramovits, MD, a physician in the purest sense of the word, honored me with the request that I read this book and comment on it.

"Humans often seek help when in pain, thinking that any health-care provider can give them proper orientation. This may be founded on the fact that most painful events resolve by themselves; some, however, require the cause to be worked up and treated in an honest-to-good way. This book directs patients so they avoid falling into the hands of quacks offering healing through esoteric therapies that may delay proper treatment, endanger them, or make their situation unsolvable.

"I specialize in cancer surgery, so I am keenly aware of the importance of finding the correct physician as early as possible for the best chance of a cure. Dr. Abramovits provides an efficient algorithm for that.

"This is a much-needed book for all to read and avoid the disastrous consequences of seeking care at the wrong place. I firmly believe that this book will SAVE LIVES!"

—Eduardo Souchon, MD, FACS, Professor of Surgery, University of Texas, McGovern Medical School, Houston, TX, UT Health Dean's Excellence Teaching Award 2005-8-9-10-11-12-13 (Retired 2015), UT Health Surgical Chief Resident's Award 2005/6-2007-9, Ralph E. Ligon Award (Humanitarian, Master Surgeon, Mentor of Medical Residents and Students) 2009–13

Preface

This book is meant to save people from the consequences of obtaining health care from the wrong providers.

Even highly educated people may be misinformed or confused about terms like "provider," "doctor," "board-certified," and many others, about which I explain or warn as we proceed.

How dare I assume that many of you, my readers, may be misinformed?

Well, because not a day goes by in which I am not disgusted, angered, repulsed, or offended by the hoaxes I see perpetrated on the public, by the media, and even in places where patient care may be provided.

If I were not a medical doctor, I, too, would be fooled by the daunting number of medical falsehoods or "fake news" that is sometimes given subliminally and other times shamelessly in your face.

They are all around me: in car wash magazines, newspapers and tabloids, subway posters, freeway billboards, and most notably, on the radio, television, and the web.

I see some in "infomercials," delivered by now-called "influencers" (of "idiotensers," of course), throughout the web and other media. Some people are lazy and prefer to have others do their thinking.

In an after-midnight thirty-minute-long infomercial, which I consider a crock of fecal matter, two, no-doubt, quacks (medical charlatans), one identified in the subtitles as "doctor and master herbalist," the other I forget (but it is irrelevant), claiming that over two million people have already bought the colon cleansers they push. For your sake, I hope you were not another of the likely millions of buyers who have fallen into their trap.

There are many, many other examples of intentionally deceptive, if not downright unethical, if not criminal, false advertising, from which the public seems not adequately protected by the proper authorities, such as the Food and Drug Administration (FDA), the Federal Trade Commission (FTC), consumer groups, the police, the Federal Bureau of Investigations (FBI), and the like.

These ads include ones for creams with names like "body X on," where the X substitutes for a part of the body, like "temple-on" to relieve headaches or "anus-on" to relieve pain in the piles (I just invented the latter). In small print, most of those should say "not proven to work by the FDA" or "homeopathic."

Falsely advertised products may also include "serums" that fix dark circles under the eyes and fade decades of sun-caused skin aging, as well as ones that erase brown spots and wrinkles quickly and permanently, sometimes by the grace of "particles." Cellulite-reducing gels, colored capsules, powders, or chewy cubes promise a quick and persistent return to bygone abilities and energy, normalizing blood pressure, fixing erectile dysfunction, correcting visual or hearing issues, and solving memory lapses—you name it.

Many people do not read the labels on those products, trusting that government agencies intended to protect them, like the FDA or the FTC, regulate such products on their behalf (which I believe they would like to do but lack sufficient authority to do).

Some scamming products are sold at gas stations (next to the cashier or the sushi), "health" food stores, car washes, and more, often near the sexual enhancers, in little bottles, colored capsules, pills, and so on. "Location, location, location!"

How about those magnetic bracelets for balance issues or arthritis, which the Cuban Shark laughed off as useless (well-based, mind you)? And those insoles that change color as they suck out one's toxins through the sweaty feet, hence "purifying" the body? Or the older weight-loss pills, some of which were recalled after reports of heart attacks and strokes. The newer ones work remarkably well, albeit not without risks, and when adequately prescribed by a doctor who is not pushing them on TV at bargain prices.

How about the "nutraceutical" promotions using a guy with the smile of an imbecile for "male enhancement"? Fortunately, their commercial seems off the air. I would not want to meet any women he picked up through the ad and, I bet, displeased.

The owner of one of those products was sentenced to twenty-five years in jail for scamming in this way.

How about the so-called "influencers" on the web, with millions of followers, giving medical advice on various conditions and diseases about what they "don't know diddly." Notice that they also add to the promo, in small print or too fast to be readable: "This is not medical advice, nor should it be construed as it..." (because they fear penalties from a government agency).

A joke among medical doctors is that "Dr. Google kills everybody," likely because they always consider the legal implications of a possible death due to the advice it gives out.

Look at a pair of colored capsules peddled by a "doctor" who claims to have attended medical school. Maybe he did, briefly, but he likely didn't graduate, as he became a chiropractor.

I bet that a woman in one of the ads, who claims to be fifty-two years old, suggests she looks younger (haha!) and asserts she is a "family medicine physician." However, she may be a fraudster who is not a medical doctor (MD) or osteopathic doctor (DO), as neither designation appeared in the ad. I couldn't find her on any state medical board or even on Google. (Red flag!) Another woman in a related ad hints at being a "physical medicine specialist" and credits her inordinate energy to the ad capsules; I bet she never attended medical or osteopathic school. In such cases, I firmly believe the medical board of their respective state should suspend their licenses for impersonation. A third woman identifies herself as a "therapist," not an MD or DO.

Indeed, none of the initial three apparent "doctors" or "physicians" in the colored capsule ads graduated from medical schools (one or two are chiropractors, another an optometrist, others who knows what?). Did you notice it? Probably not. Marketeers (a derogatory term for marketers) know how to disguise falsehoods.

In 2019, the FDA sent the chiropractor a warning letter, which I quote as follows: "The inspection and our review of your product labeling revealed serious violations of the Federal Food, Drug, and Cosmetic Act and applicable regulations."

How about some chewy, must-be fructose-rich root crystals offering to deliver, using a TV personality, "amazing energy"? Placebo effect? Doesn't plain old sugar do that? Just add a vitamin or two and make a claim.

I recently saw a TV ad saying (paraphrasing), "Hair loss in male pattern baldness has to do with the enzyme that converts testosterone into dihydrotestosterone (DHT), which is a hundred times more potent." This factoid was immediately followed by "Our shampoo makes hair grow!" implying that it does through the enzyme. But that is not the case (red flag!). There is no shampoo approved by the FDA that indeed grows hair. Maybe it appears so by thickening the strands by coating or hydrating them temporarily—a half-truth, which is the same as a half-lie, yet many don't get it on the fly. I also do not recommend those improvised by compounding pharmacies.

If you bought any of the abovementioned products or services, you fell for deceptive ads and were, sadly, bamboozled. (Like I did when I bought a fake of a famous Peter Max painting, so don't feel lonely.) I bet you did not receive any of the promised benefits, took a considerable risk, and wasted what could have been precious money. I'm sorry! You were duped, deceived, and bamboozled.

And, if you thought you got something good out of them, you probably figured out what the "placebo" effect" feels like. In the long run, most fooled customers stop taking those things because of side effects or dwindling perceived benefits.

You may want to know that marketers expect buyers to return no more than about 5 percent of what they received and are unhappy with, even when ads offer warranties, like "your money back," for dissatisfaction.

Quite often, after raking in millions of dollars, products that don't work at all or don't do their job well enough go the way of the dodo, although by then, fly-by-nighters who know how to exploit the public made their killing and took it to the bank.

If you happen to have been one of the millions who bought books by Kevin Trudeau titled *Natural Cures "They" Don't Want You to Know About*, my apologies for not writing this guide sooner; thus, preventing many of you from falling for his ads. Or from those of other scammers.

Learn this right now (it is imperative): Sums of anecdotes do not make acceptable, reliable, scientific clinical data. Doubt all ads that use anecdotes or personal accounts (like "it worked for me, so it should work for you too") to convince you to buy a product or service are a well-known marketing trick that violates the scientific method we "real doctors" require and demand.

Even lousy products, marketed cleverly (if unethically), can become bestsellers.

Beware, even if the storyteller is a likable famous person (an old sports hero or politician), a puppy, or a cartoon character, you may become the victim of a trap, bamboozled.

I want my readers to question marketers' ethics and tactics in commercials, particularly those on expensive and repetitive television ads. Never overlook the saying, "If it sounds too good to be true, it probably is." Please write it down a thousand times so you won't forget like I did when I bought a fake painting by Peter Max.

In an ad for a cancer treatment center, I noticed (discreetly mentioned) that they collaborate with alternative, complementary, and integrative medicine providers (red flag!)—as if that were a good thing—and that they have appointments "available now." (another red flag!)

Many commercials resemble the pressure from the proverbial car salesman, who does whatever it takes to make a potential client commit to something that might obligate one to buy a car—signing a piece of paper before leaving the dealership's showroom. In the case of health care, never succumb to pressure over getting the best possible doctor, product, or service. My mission with this guide is to inform and thus empower patients to refuse mediocre medicine or be bamboozled.

Be mindful and not attracted to buy anti-aging "serums," like if they are non-stick frying pans or vacuums, confidently saying "free to the first 300 callers in your area" repeatedly over months, which doesn't make sense. (Red flag!) Nor are products discounted if you buy "within the next thirty or so minutes" repeatedly, which doesn't make sense. (Red flag!)

The point is: Question all commercials! Scrutinize them in precise detail, or they will win you over. Don't "impulse buy!"

Read the tiny print in blurry fonts stating something like "the FDA has not verified these claims," and don't trust half, even if they use phrases like "university-conducted study" or "a double-blind, placebo-controlled study." You may need to pause TV commercials to read the tiny print.

Be careful with clinics that, even if "run by doctors," offer quasi-miracles. For example, injections and prescriptions that are "only sold here" (red flag!) to lose weight, tone up, and make people in their seventies look like they are in their forties, with lots of hair and great erections (wink-wink). A newer example is rejuvenating topicals containing peptides (particles of proteins or amino acids) developed explicitly for men.

Watch out for ads that peddle contraptions or shots that make penises enlarge, heal arthritis, and reduce or delay the need for joint surgery by injecting your own healing cells (their success vs. failure and complications are still under investigation, but one wouldn't know it judging from ads).

How many more times will you fall for diet ads offered in "health" magazines next to supermarket cashiers, on TV ads, and elsewhere? Another thousand?

What is the medical training of your "life coach"? I can see those characters employed by stuck-ups in sports, trophy wives, movie actors, or drug dealers with money to throw, but not you or me. Where do "life coaches" get such a degree? At

Needless Markup, Goodmen's, Bloommer's, Sak's? You already know what life coaches tell you to do: eat fresh fruits and vegetables, exercise, don't smoke, don't drink alcohol (that's the latest), don't do drugs, what shoes to buy, what color clothing goes best against your skin, and other bull. And then they'll send you a bill.

Here is another piece of advice: Be cautious of medicine ads or labels that use the term "support": "supports brain function" (memory loss, fogginess, and how is any of this measured?), "supports immune systems" in combating colds, influenza, COVID-19, and other viral diseases, "supports eye function," or "supports the prostate, liver, kidneys, heart, and vascular system, including varicose veins" and everything else.

The brain is adequately supported by the base of the skull, the prostate by the pelvis, the eyes by their sockets, and so forth. Did you grasp the point? Most support for organs, systems, and functions comes from a proper diet, exercise, muscles, and bones, rather than from pills, but you already knew that (and without a life coach).

Statistically valid comparators (such as real life, placebo, other pills, etc.) are rarely used in advertisements, often misquoted, or intentionally concealed, which violates evidence-based medicine (EBM).

Statisticians who work for marketers should be exposed and made to feel embarrassed when misrepresenting or hiding the "truth in advertising," fostering fake news, or using half-truths (or half-lies, remember?). Other employees of marketing agencies should tattle tell on them. But wouldn't that be biting the hand that feeds them?

The proliferation of clinics, urgent care (UC) facilities, and stand-alone emergency rooms (ERs) conveniently located in stores, pharmacies, airports, strip malls, and more- operated not by MDs or DOs but by mid-medically-educated providers such as NPs or PAs, who possess limited and questionable knowledge and are often not supervised by an actual physician on the premises—should concern everyone.

Judging by the number of UCs and ERs popping up everywhere, they must be gold mines. I will leave that issue for a later chapter.

I may be powerless to amend most of the issues mentioned above as they are political. I am merely an MD, not a congressman or a Supreme Court justice (too busy with dealings belonging to church and family—or on free trips). However, I should have enough power to educate my readers on choosing a good doctor for themselves and their loved ones and how to blow bad ones out of the water.

Even the FDA, the FTC, and other powerful-sounding government agencies meant to protect the public too often seem incapable of fighting for adequate access to good health care. Maybe (like the police), they should be given more authority. They, too, may be victims of misrepresentation, media manipulation, and twisting. For example, advertisers may make claims like "FDA-registered" or "FDA-cleared" in ways that cause consumers to erroneously infer that the FDA "approved" them.

"FDA-cleared" means not much more than proven not unsafe enough for the public to purchase at their own risk (like some painkillers or birth control pills) and is usable in self-diagnosable conditions such as joint pain, wrinkles, or hair loss. It does not imply that the product will work for the condition claimed!

If a device or medication is proven effective and safe, the FDA will identify it as "FDA-approved." (If nothing else from this chapter, remember the word: "approved" used correctly.)

Merchants sell contraptions they tell you are "FDA-cleared." Examples include "hair-growing" red-light helmets, blue-light or other color face masks for acne and aging, joint and muscle pain, kinesiology straps, vegan and mechanical sexual enhancers, weight-loss pills, some that may later be recalled, and so on.

In short, look for "approved," not for "registered" or "cleared," if what you want is something proven to work while being safe to use.

Believe it or not, despite its many problems, the best medical care is available in the United States. However, one has to figure out how to find it, and that may require quite a bit of help. I hope to provide plenty of it with this guide.

Choosing the ideal doctor or medical facility for an individual can be problematic. It is for that reason I wrote this book.

Many marketers are competent at diverting patients from good toward wrong "doctors" through misinformation, half-lies, and other forms of bamboozling.

Politically influenced documentaries, such as *Sicko* by Michael Moore, suggest (accidentally, I hope) that patients can get better care in Cuba than in the United States of America—tell that to Hugo Chavez, the former president-cum-dictator of Venezuela, who chose cancer care in a Havana hospital over MD Anderson Cancer Center in Houston, Texas, or Memorial Hospital in New York, and quickly died. I wonder where Chavez or Moore would go nowadays.

Going to quacks (medical imposters, charlatans, and scammers) for health care is likely to result in delays in obtaining the proper attention, and it could be costly, frustrating, and, ultimately, dangerous to the point of lethal.

Quacks are pretty clever at utilizing the media to lure patients in, so beware of their marketing ploys.

Still, as many can be identified and exposed, they can be avoided and repudiated. Thus, the public can be protected from quackery.

Those reading this book will learn how to identify and skip the quacks and crooks in the following chapters.

As the front cover suggests, this guide is intended to provide some of the advice and tools needed to locate this country's highest levels of medical excellence. It offers tips on minimizing suffering and the waste of precious dollars on ineffective health-care providers and the inappropriate treatments they propose. However, it is all based on my beliefs and opinions.

To the best of my abilities, I wrote this guide objectively and transparently, providing references and recommended readings from respectable sources to support most observations and quotes. However, I must alert you of the inevitable tainting resulting from my experiences and personal philosophy about health care. (caveat emptor.)

The book is meant to be free from political or, better said, partisan influences, as I belong to no party, although, judging by the loads of polluting correspondence I get from them, someone may think I do to theirs.

It must be made clear that this guide does not provide advice on personal or individual medical matters, and no part of it should be construed for that purpose.

I state the above not only to avoid or minimize my risk of being sued by one of you, as this happens so frequently in our overrepresented society, even to "ham sandwiches," but also because the best medical practice occurs only within the realm of individualized care—the exclusive result of happy and healthy patient-doctor relationships.

Surely, there will be critics and detractors, particularly those providers who may find their trade negatively represented (not intentionally), exposed, and hurt in their pockets. I welcome their constructive opinions; as I learn from valid ones, I will use them in revised editions.

I already feel the outrage of iridologists, as well as of practitioners of Reiki, Rolfing, and functional medicine, colonic cleansers, chiropractors, chelators, homeopaths, and a myriad of other versions of complementary, alternative, and integrative health care (CAIH) providers.

I do not wish nor intend to belittle or offend valuable healthcare providers like nurse practitioners and physician assistants, but that could tacitly happen when comparing their education to that of MDs and DOs. What they may be are mid-medically educated providers of healthcare (MEPs).

Finally, it was inevitable not to frame the book within my feelings regarding the progression or regression of medical care in the US. The latter is a sensation that older patients and peers notice, but it is one to which young resident physicians and medical students are waking up and adapting because they do not know better.

Experienced and mature yet still practicing "real" doctors like me, and patients are aware that current health care is inadequate, expensive, and deteriorating despite remarkable technological and pharmaceutical advances.

Ah, one more point: English is my second language (Spanish is my first); hence, you may often notice grammatical faux pas that escaped me, linguists, and editors, including those based on artificial intelligence (AI). In the words of the famous philosopher (and comedian) Steve Martin, "Excuuuse meee!!"

For entertaining purposes and readability, I write somewhat colloquially but clean of foul language (more like Seinfeld and Nate Bargatze—pardon to them), sarcastically or translating, and with a (sick?) sense of humor that not all understand. If you dislike my style, please send me your opinions, corrections, and suggestions for the next edition, and then make the most of the "meat" of the text.

Another point: I wrote this guide without assistance from the tools AI provides, only an editor tool, which I fought a lot. I may use them in future editions, although towards the end, I used Grammarly to survey for errors; I corrected over a thousand suggestions but left lots as they were.

Now, let's find you (and everyone) some good doctors.

We understand that MDs and DOs do not have a monopoly on the term doctor, nor should they. We do not need or want it for ego or monetary reasons. We have better reasons, like the joy of making patients better. However, we earned it much more deservingly than others who (mis)use it.

References and Recommended Reading

1. *American Greed*, Episode 33, "Sexual Performance Pill / Kirk Wright," aired April 14, 2010, on CNBC.
2. "Natural Cures 'They' Don't Want You to Know About," *Wikipedia*, https://en.wikipedia.org/wiki/Natural_Cures_%22They%22_Don%27t_Want_You_to_Know_About.
3. Liz Szabo, "How to Guard Against a Quack," *USA Today*, June 18, 2013, https://www.usatoday.com/story/news/nation/2013/06/18/how-to-spot-a-quack/2429471/.
4. "Protect Desperate Patients from the Houston Cancer Quack," *Skeptical Inquirer. 2014;37(2).*

Glossary

ABMS	American Board of Medical Specialties
ABPS	American Board of Physician Specialties
ABPS	American Board of Plastic Surgery
ACGME	Accreditation Council for Graduate Medical Education
ASPS	American Society of Plastic Surgeons
AMA	American Medical Association
AOA	American Osteopathic Association
APsyA	American Psychoanalytic Association
AI	Artificial Intelligence
EBM	Evidence-Based Medicine
CAM	Complementary and Alternative Medicine
CAIH	Complementary, Alternative and Integrative Healthcare
DC	Doctor of Chiropractic
DO	Doctor of Osteopathy
MD	Medical Doctor
FDA	Food and Drug Administration
FTC	Federal Trade Commission
FM	Functional Medicine
FP	Family Practitioner

DDS	Doctor of Dental Surgery
DPM	Doctor of Podiatric Medicine
DT	Dental Therapists
OD	Optometry Doctor
DVM	Doctor of Veterinary Medicine
MA	Medical Assistant
PA	Physician Assistant
LVN	Licensed Vocational Nurse
RN	Registered Nurse
NP	Nurse Practitioner
NA	Nurse Anesthetist
MEP	Mid-educated Provider
APP	Advanced Practice Provider
NPP	Non-Physician Practitioner
ND	Naturopathic Doctor
PT	Physical Therapist
RD	Registered Dietitian
PhD	Philosophical Doctor
PsyD	Psychology Doctor
PsyPhD	Philosophical Doctor in Psychology
GPA	Grade Point Average
MCAT	Medical College Admission Test
ECFMG	Educational Council for Foreign Medical Graduates
NB	National Boards
MOC	Maintenance of Certification
USMLE	United States Medical Licensing Examination
FTC	Federal Trade Commission

NIH	National Institutes of Health
NCCIH	National Center for Complementary and Integrative Health
US	United States
USA	United States of America
UK	United Kingdom
ER	Emergency Room
UC	Urgent Care
ICU	Intensive Care Unit
SCAM	So-Called Alternative Medicine

When a -C is added to the suffix (PA-C or MA-C, for example), it implies Certified.

Who Is a Doctor (Dr.)? And What Is a Physician?

With this book, I intend to expose why the medical care many get in the US sometimes falls below expectations, particularly regarding who provides it.

"Doctor" is not the exclusive domain of any given group. Yet, it is an excellent term for propagandizing oneself, particularly when one is not an actual medical or osteopathic school graduate.

In today's market, anyone can label themselves a "doctor" and establish a "clinic" or "hospital." Isn't that absurd? This phenomenon explains the prevalence of terms like "windshield doctors," "carpet doctors," "dirt doctors," "shoe hospitals," "lock doctors," "glass doctors," "car clinics," and more.

Photographs can be "doctored" using AI tools. Information technologists (IT) may work using "disk doctors," people can drink "Dr. Pepper" and listen to "Dr. Dré." And so on.

As a dermatologist, I considered myself the quintessential "itch doctor" or "scar doctor" until I discovered products called "scratch or dent doctors" at auto parts stores. These are sold over the counter without a prescription!

I have even seen "car dermatologists" on the road. I also noticed a "pipe doctor" truck; at first, I thought it was for prostate enlargement or constipation, but it wasn't. It was a plumber's advertisement. (I bet urologists, gastroenterologists, and colon and rectal surgeons don't appreciate the joke.)

I imagine there could be "truck proctologists" (you know, for the exhaust); I discovered a "Lock Dr." who presumably works with safes or chastity belts. There's even a "Dr. Gold" who sounds like a nice Jewish dermatologist in Nashville, TN, but was a jeweler in Dallas.

These so-called "doctors" have nothing to do with medicine and are easy to spot, identify, and laugh at because they pose no danger or concern to society. Instead, I find their ads to be cute and clever.

Problems arise when people in health care portray themselves as "doctors" when they are not—at least not medical doctors (MDs) or doctors of osteopathy (DOs).

The title "doctor" has been usurped and misappropriated! The public can no longer assume it belongs to someone who has earned an MD or DO degree from a medical school. (I'll elaborate.)

It is easy to be misled into believing that chiropractors (DC), who refer to themselves as "doctors of chiropractic" or "chiropractic physicians," optometrists (ODs), who call themselves "eye doctors" and podiatrists (DPMs), who identify as "foot doctors"; among others, graduated from "medical school," when they did not, at least not from a program that grants physician MD or DO degrees.

These "doctors" often claim to have attended some form of "medical school," but they cannot honestly assert that it is equivalent to those that train MDs or DOs—because it isn't.

For example, no matter how valuable and important they may be in medical care, foot doctors receive a DPM degree from a podiatry school rather than an MD or DO degree in foot and ankle medicine. In contrast, orthopedists complete medical school and can treat diseases of the foot as well as other parts of the body. Thus, podiatrists' scope of practice is currently limited to the foot and ankle (see the chapter on podiatry), while a specialized MD or DO does not face such limitations.

The press often refers to our former First Lady as "Dr. Jill Biden." Her "doctorate" is in education, not at the PhD level or within the field of medicine. The reason the press addresses her as "Doctor" Biden is intriguing, confusing, and may reflect brown-nosing or simply ignorance. Even Whoopi mistakenly suggested that Jill should become the next surgeon general, and when corrected, she appropriately apologized to her audience.

This book aims to address that type of issue.

Other "health care providers" who do not undergo physician (MD or DO) training include most or all "functional" or "naturopathic" doctors (FMDs or NDs), physician assistants (PAs), or physician associates (as they now prefer to be called), nurse practitioners (NPs), certified nurse-midwives (CNMs), nurse anesthetists (CRNAs), all advanced practice providers (APPs) or non-physician providers (NPPs), homeopaths, acupuncturists, psychologists and therapists, chiropractors (DCs), and others that the reader will learn about in later chapters.

In the US, only two types of medical school graduates are legally permitted to practice "real" medicine independently. These schools confer MD or DO degrees.

No other healthcare providers undergo those types of medical schooling, and their graduates should not attempt to present themselves as physicians.

The education of chiropractors, optometrists, podiatrists, PAs, NPs, and others differs significantly from what I refer to as "real" physicians and surgeons. MDs and DOs are regulated by distinct laws that govern their respective trades.

In other words, when chiropractors, optometrists, podiatrists, NPPs, psychotherapists, functional medicine providers, and similar "providers" graduate, they do not become MDs or DOs and cannot legally identify themselves as such. The degrees they have earned are limited to their area of study.

The dental school exemplifies this situation. It offers "real" doctorates in dental surgery (DDS) or dental medicine (DMD), which, although equivalent, are distinct from MD or DO degrees. Again, this difference does not diminish the value of their medical education; they are the professionals I rely on for my dental care.

If "providers"—regardless of how "advanced" they may be in their field—do not hold an MD or DO degree, they must never portray or identify themselves as doctors of medicine or surgery, under penalty of law. Ethically, they should clarify that they are not "doctors" to prevent misinterpretation as physicians by their patients, even if they have obtained a PhD or other doctorate in nursing, physician assistance, nurse anesthesia, psychology, pharmacy, or a similar field. Yet, some do not.

Generally, while caring for patients and claiming to be doctors, "providers" who are not MDs or DOs must specify the field of their doctorates and inform patients when their degrees are not in medicine. Failing to disclose or clarify that their doctorates are not in medicine can be considered intentionally misleading and a violation of ethics if not the law, which could result in a penalty or revocation of their license. Yet they rarely do so and often get away with it.

MDs and DOs dislike being grouped under the label "providers," just as NPPs dislike being referred to as "mid-levels" or medically mid-educated practitioners. The term "provider" carries an ugly past; it is what Jewish doctors were called in Nazi concentration camps under Hitler's orders.

Nurse practitioners (NPs) have applied for the right to prescribe medications without direct supervision by MDs or DOs and have successfully obtained this privilege in some states (a significant mistake, in my opinion). Physician assistants (PAs) seek the same right (which would be another mistake). They believe they are at least equal to NPs.

MDs and DOs express grievances when NPPs receive practice privileges not via the study of medicine but through influencing members of Congress, a result of lobbying that may be achieved by promising election or reelection votes. How does that sound to you? To me, it sounds like corruption—something Congress has many of us used to.

NPs and PAs can obtain PhDs or "professional doctorates" in their fields (DNP, DMS), even online, without touching a single patient. Such programs allow graduates to refer to themselves as doctors despite not being doctors of medicine. I think this intends to blur lines and allow many to take advantage, if not pleasure, in the resulting confusion.

Don't count on mid-levels, with (or without) doctorates, to make things clear to patients voluntarily and spontaneously. They love it when they call them "doctors" and rarely prompt themselves to say that their doctorate is not in medicine.

Another example of usurpation is the petition by pharmacists to be recognized as "primary healthcare providers" (implying the ability to prescribe), similar to other NPPs. Some states have granted certain advanced pharmacists prescribing privileges, albeit with limitations; these include Paxlovid™ for COVID-19, as well as vaccines for shingles, influenza, and other infections; medications such as Tamiflu™ for the flu, and potentially, if not already, birth control and abortion pills. The prescribing of Paxlovid™ by pharmacists was intended solely to address a public health emergency—however, once the cats are out of the bag…

Further attempts to encroach upon the field of medicine are exemplified by the determination of podiatrists and optometrists. They seek to broaden the scope of their practices to align more closely with that of MDs and DOs. Recently, even optometrists were permitted to prescribe certain eye drops. Turf expansions often occur in Congress rather than schools providing education and training.

Why is the term "doctor" seemingly so desirable?

Because it allows non-medical doctors (of the wrong kind, if you ask me, and providers with inferiority complexes) to market themselves to gullible, poorly informed consumers for ego trips, to impress chicks, to attain monetary aspirations, and more, all without putting in the effort, investment, and time it takes to go through a real medical school.

Why is the term doctor so easy to usurp?

Because of a lack of adequate legislation and enforcement.

As many of you believe, know, or at least sense, lobbying is a form of legalized corruption susceptible to voter power. I may be repeating this intentionally for good reasons.

For instance, the number of optometrists is 2.5 times greater than that of ophthalmologists (likely a realistic figure provided by the Department of Labor); regardless of what may be best for the public, in whose favor do you think the balance will shift among those in Congress running for reelection?

How can chiropractors—who do not attend medical school—rightfully call themselves "doctors" in chiropractic, "chiropractic physicians," or, as I saw printed on the door of a nearby office, "doctor in orthopedic chiropractic" and "board-certified in sports medicine"? (In my opinion, the latter represents an inappropriate, unethical, and possibly illegal misuse of the term "board-certified.")

Again, Congress or another governmental office should provide the answer. I hope these abuses will be fixed soon.

Remember that the term "board-certified" is explicitly recognized for "real" physicians by the American Board of Medical Specialties (ABMS) for MDs and by the American Osteopathic Association's (AOA) Department of Certifying Board Services for DOs. Therefore, "board-certified" is another usurped term—more on that later.

Congress's response to the chiropractor issue also applies to other providers, including most alternative medicine doctors, complementary medicine doctors, integrative medicine doctors, holistic physicians, naturopathic physicians, and others, unless they were previously MDs or DOs who strayed from their original educational paths (which is a rare occurrence). That situation reminds me of the joke about a military guy who became a sergeant the hard way by first being a general. (drum roll.)

Some of those non-MD and non-DO individuals, as well as non-physician practitioners (NPPs), do not provide the "good medicine" they profess but rather questionable alternatives: practices that do not adhere to "evidence-based," "best-available," or "proven-effective" knowledge, failing to properly utilize the scientific method.

Returning to the chapter title question, "physician" denotes a "person legally qualified to practice medicine; a doctor of medicine who is not a surgeon." However, "not a surgeon" is outdated.

My graduation diploma from medical school in 1972–3 states "Physician and Surgeon," which somewhat acknowledges the prior definition. However, this may undervalue the MD or DO degree recipient, as they are now legally qualified to perform surgeries for which they received proper training in medical school or afterward. Therefore, I would prefer "Doctor of Medicine and Surgery."

Confused? Maddeningly so? Let me try to deconfuse you.

A lack of clarity may enable some providers to claim "doctor" and "physician." A Google search for "physician" yields various synonyms: doctor, doctor of medicine, MD, and medical practitioner. However, it also includes terms like "healer" and "physician of the soul," suggesting that the title "physician" does not necessarily imply "medical doctor."

Even the use of the title "physician," usurped or not, whether informally, intentionally, or illegally used by PAs, NPs, midwives, chiropractors, and the like, may be a misappropriation of the title, which is why they are called non-physician practitioners (NPPs)—their fault for greedy.

Confused even worse? Let's keep deconfusing you.

A recent update from the Social Security Administration regarding the definition of "physician" includes 'Doctor of Medicine and Osteopathy, Doctor of Dental Surgery or Dental Medicine, Doctor of Podiatric Medicine (with limitations), Doctor of Optometry (with limitations), and Chiropractor (with certain minimum standards),' provided that they are legally authorized by the state where the practice is located. This definition, slightly rephrased, only adds to the confusion.

Oddly, it excludes explicitly Christian Science practitioners and naturopaths. Unfortunately, some states, such as Oregon, do include naturopaths as physicians. Like so many other government attempts to fix things, this one worsened despite possible good intentions. I wonder how much that cost in dollars and votes.

The word "physician," like "doctor," needs upgrading, updating, restricting, or regulating. Perhaps what it needs is replacing.

Don't be fooled by those who call themselves "physician extenders," "assistants," or "associates." Many try to make you think they went through medical school when they didn't. They are not equally educated and cannot be equally competent. (Not even close.)

In some states, PAs have tried to replace their title of "assistant" with "associate" in an apparent attempt to fool the public further. They don't want to be perceived as assistants. If you ask some PAs who their supervising physician is, they respond that they don't need one because they are not anybody's "assistant." They now claim to be "associates." NPs are going for "partner or "collaborator."

The American Osteopathic Association (AOA) published a position statement advocating for truth in advertising, intellectual honesty, and transparency when using professional designations like "clinician" (a linguistic trick intended to deceive) in response to APRNs, PAs and other NPPs who inappropriately use the titles "doctor" or "clinician."

Professional doctorates exist in nursing practice (DNP), podiatry (DPM), optometry (OD, not to be confused with DO), pharmacy (PharmD), psychology (PsyD), and other forms of health care.

Doctorate degrees, obtained through advanced education, have existed for decades in fields such as physics, chemistry, mathematics, biology, history, and even religion. However, these types of doctorates are typically academic (such as Ph.Ds), usually take about five years, and necessitate original research, which must be presented to faculty as a dissertation. The medical professional doctorates I am addressing here do not have the same research requirements and generally have a shorter duration (although exceptions exist on both sides).

A patient once asked me for a "professional discount" (something obsolete and odd as most doctors nowadays are insured) "being that we are both doctors." I asked him what his doctorate was in. "Deity," he replied. "Who provided you with such a doctorate?" "My church," he said. I'm leaving it at that.

Regarding dentists as Doctors of Dental Surgery or Dental Medicine (DDS or DDM), their status as non-MDs or DOs does not diminish the value of their degrees or the care they provide. I visit dentists regularly, as everyone should. I also refer patients with conditions affecting the inside of the mouth for consultations, biopsies, surgeries, and other services that exceed the scope of my medical practice, and they help me greatly in these matters.

Although working in another area of medicine, dentists are my equal peers. Some practice and teach at the same medical schools I am affiliated with. However, I still check their credentials as I would with any doctor I intend to go to—like when I want to ask for recommendations from them or my medical colleagues. Be aware that in Colorado, a precedent was set that allows dental hygienists, not the dentists themselves, to inject fillers and botulinum toxin for cosmetic purposes.

In the following chapters, I outline the formative steps required to become an MD or DO and compare them to many other medical careers; this is to "deconfuse" you as much as possible so you don't get "bamboozled."

I wrote this chapter and many that follow so you can compare the degrees and knowledge among healthcare professionals, and to allow me to address how some dare to call themselves, or wish to be called, "doctors" without putting in the effort that graduating from a "real" medical school requires. All too often, this is done senselessly, unethically, and irresponsibly!

It also allows me to clarify the distinctions among MDs, DOs, and other types of providers for my readers. I encourage you to be mindful of this for your own sake and that of your loved ones.

Start by searching for the suffix "MD" or "DO" following the name of your "doctor" (even if the prefix "Dr." shows up before their name, such omission should alert you that the provider has not gone through medical school and could be an imposter).

As physicians' earnings continue to decline, some MDs and DOs feel compelled to expand and diversify their practices. Many offer services such as injecting botulinum toxins and fillers, for which dermatologists and plastic surgeons are more appropriately trained. Gynecologists and dentists now commonly offer such services, and they may delegate them to weekend-trained mid-levels or those so-called "nurse injectors," many having minimal knowledge and experience in facial anatomy, physiology, pharmacology, and the like. Such delegates may be ill-equipped to manage the resulting complications. (Buyer beware!)

Some doctor offices nowadays retail cosmetics, low-power red light lasers and LED helmets, and combs (supposedly to grow hair); depilate armpits and pubic areas; remove tattoos, bleach anuses; peddle vitamins, and even housewares through pyramid schemes; retail exercise equipment, sell (magical?) workout strips, bandages, and other accouterments to have an extra source of revenue. (How tragic!)

Other doctors often take on second jobs, such as spa supervisors (often remotely) and insurance company consultants, where they' filter" (if not block) services and medications recommended by their peers to patients they have never seen, among other roles. Some may even serve as advisors to malpractice lawyers or medical private equity firms, like those undermining private practices by intruding into the business aspects of patient care.

Adding to the myriad stressors of our medical practices are concerns about giving special attention to severely ill patients, unmet income or salary expectations, the need to pay rent and wages to ancillary employees, legal personnel issues arising from impositions by human resources departments, especially for those working with private equities (PEs) or other financial organizations), governmental audits, and much more.

For all that and more, I don't understand why the MD or DO title is so coveted by non-physicians, particularly by complementary, alternative, and integrative healthcare (CAIH) practitioners. I presume ignorance and greed.

If NPPs want to get rich quickly, they invade the turf of the wrong profession! This is not because we are "protecting the dollar" or "defending our turf." It is because this is a matter of public health. Physicians are patients, too. We want the best care for our patients, our families, and ourselves.

As one of my sons once said when I suggested he attend medical school, "Not a chance…you work too hard, earn little, and carry too much worry." Judging by his current income from his work in wealth management, he was right. I tell you, youngsters in medicine have a bleak economic future.

Becoming a crook in many other professions is so much simpler and more profitable.

Impersonating doctors for riches is simply risky, abject stupidity.

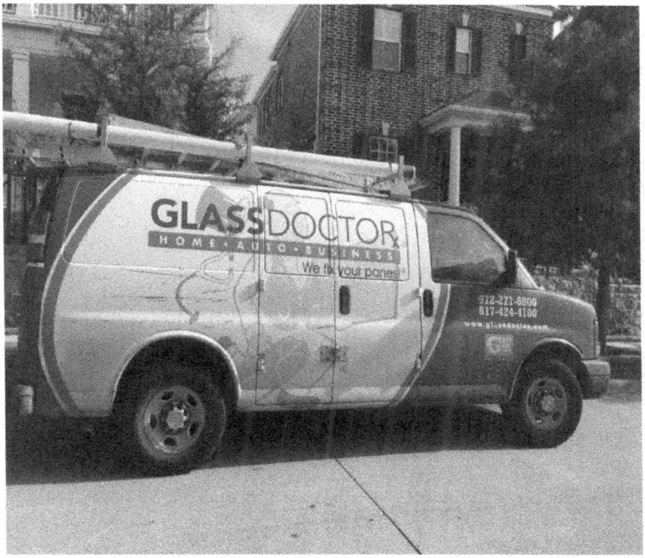
GLASSDOCTOR
HOME • AUTO • BUSINESS
We fix your panes!
972-271-8800
817-424-4100

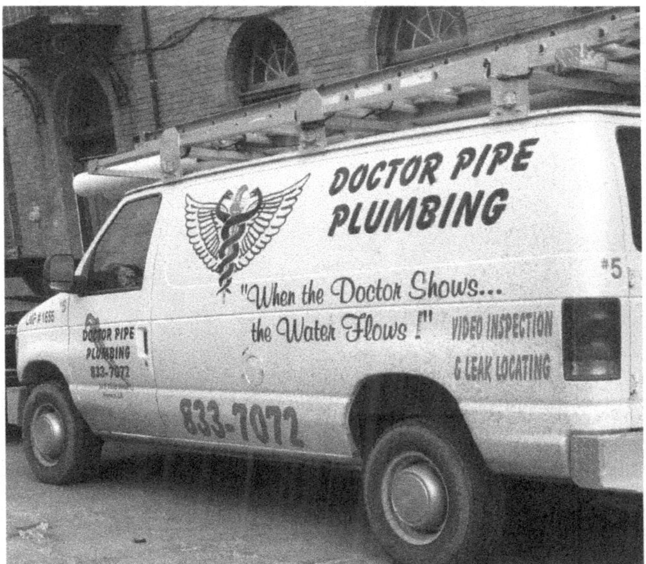
DOCTOR PIPE
PLUMBING
"When the Doctor Shows...
the Water Flows!"
VIDEO INSPECTION
& LEAK LOCATING
#5
833-7072
DOCTOR PIPE
PLUMBING
833-7072

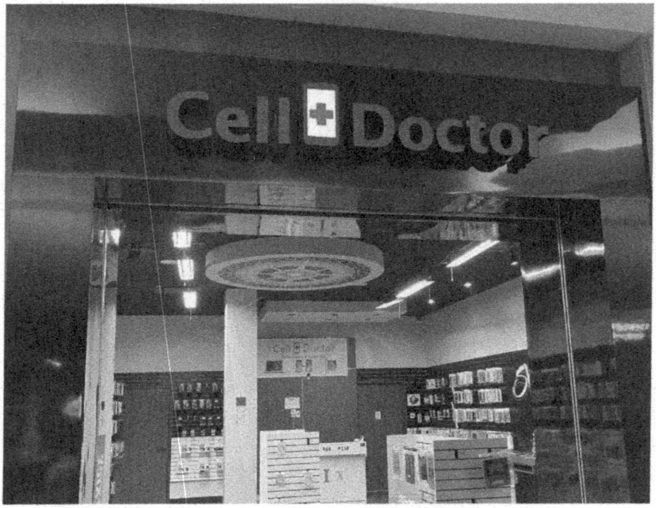
Cell Doctor

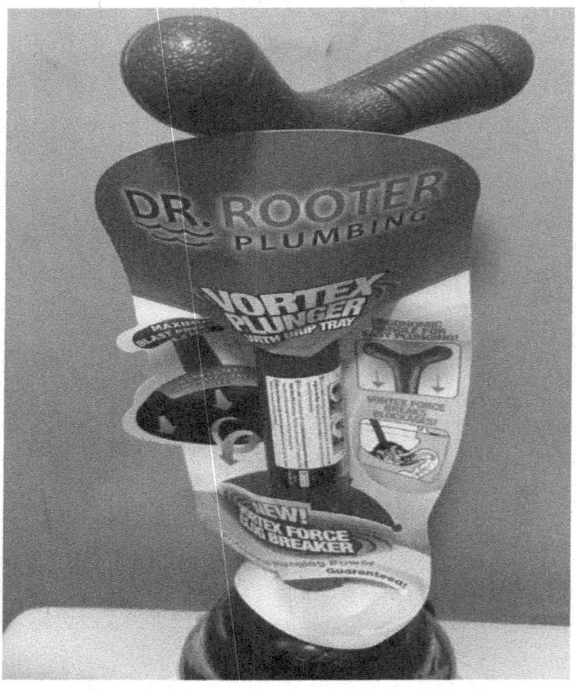
DR. ROOTER
PLUMBING
VORTEX PLUNGER
NEW!
VORTEX FORCE CLOG BREAKER
Guaranteed!

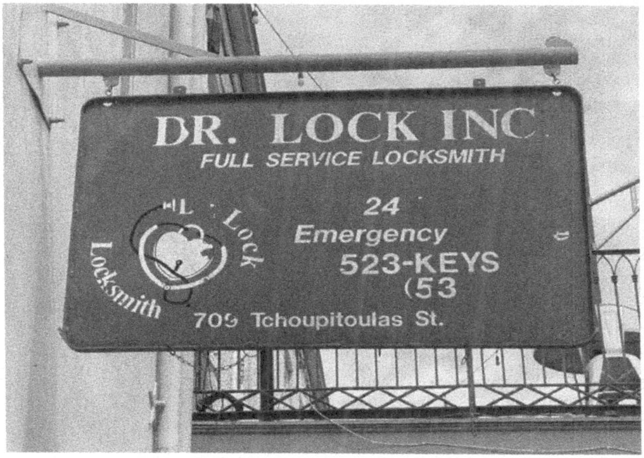
DR. LOCK INC
FULL SERVICE LOCKSMITH
Locksmith
24
Emergency
523-KEYS
(53
709 Tchoupitoulas St.

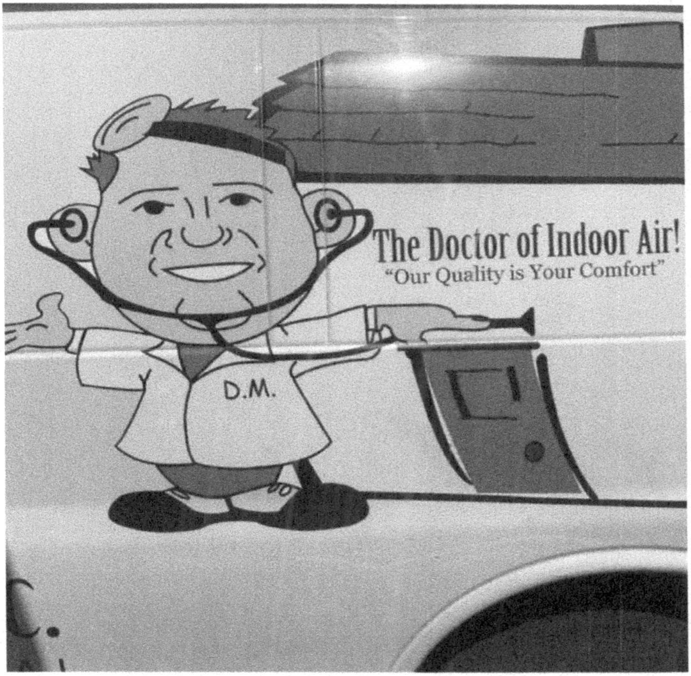
The Doctor of Indoor Air!
"Our Quality is Your Comfort"
D.M.

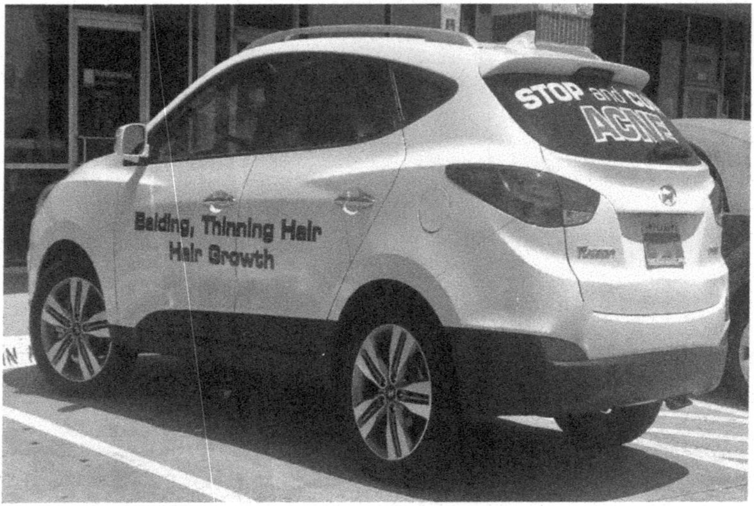
STOP and
ACNE
Balding, Thinning Hair
Hair Growth

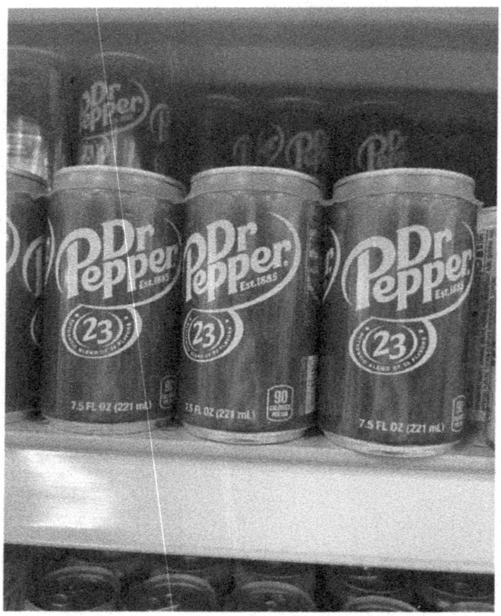
Dr Pepper
Est.1885
23
7.5 FL OZ (221 mL)

References and Recommended Readings

1. Alex Evans, "Prescribing Authority for Pharmacists: Rules and Regulations by State," July 22, 2022, https://www.goodrx.com/hcp/pharmacists/prescriber-authority-for-pharmacists.
2. "Social Security Program Operations Manual System (POMS)," Social Security Administration, October 27, 2022, https://secure.ssa.gov/poms.nsf/lnx/0600401295.
3. "Pharmacy Prescriptions: Who May Issue a Prescription?" Texas State Board of Pharmacy, accessed November 18, 2022, https://www.pharmacy.texas.gov/consumer/broch4.asp.
4. Jeffrey Lehman and Shirelle Phelps, *West's Encyclopedia of American Law* (Thomson/Gale 2005).
5. Adam Rubenfire, "Some N.Y. Nurse Practitioners to Be Freed of Doc Supervision in 2015," Modern Healthcare, http://modern-healthcare.com/article/20141230/NEWS/312309974.
6. TMA wins victory in legal battle with podiatrists. http://www.texmed.org/Template.aspx?id-17261.
7. Stephanie Innes, "Pharmacists Looking for a New Label," *Arizona Daily Star*, January 15, 2012, http://azstarnet.com/business/local/pharmacists-looking-for-a-new-label/article_cc80cf7c-7b83-52ec-a312-53f656e65baa.html.
8. AOA Staff, "AOA Statement on Physician-Led Care, Physician Assistant Title Change, and Non-Physician Clinician Use of the Title 'Doctor.'" American Osteopathic Association, May 28, 2021, https://osteopathic.org/2021/05/28/aoa-statement-on-physician-led-care-physician-assistant-title-change-and-non-physician-clinician-use-of-the-title-doctor/.
9. Salvatore Mangione, Brian F. Mandell, and Stephen G. Post, "The Language Game: We Are Physicians, Not Providers," *The American Journal of Medicine*, vol. 134,12 (2021): 1444–1446. https://doi.org/10.1016/j.amjmed.2021.06.031.

What Is Medicine?

Medicine is the practice of maintaining and restoring health. It entrusts medical doctors with the responsibility to prevent and treat diseases, cure patients, alleviate their suffering when a cure is impossible, and avert suffering and death.

In dictionaries, a patient (not a client, mind you) requires or receives medical treatment or care from a physician or hospital (but you knew that—I adhere to certain definitions for legal reasons).

To diagnose and treat, doctors rely on interviews with patients, their relatives, caregivers, and anyone close to them and their environment. They also draw knowledge from public health issues, physical exams, laboratory studies, and tests. Hmm, doesn't that sound holistic?

Medicine is regarded as an admixture of science and art, where the scientific component and AI progressively supersede the art, quite likely to everybody's benefit. Science, overtaking the art of practicing through evidence-based medicine (EBM), technological advances, and whatever comes next (like advanced AI), should lead to optimal and realistic patient care paradigms.

AI-assisted computers should replace physicians; in my opinion, the sooner, the better. This will help eliminate quackery. Neither you nor your children should have to read books like this in the near future, but for now, it would be wiser to continue reading this one. AI is unlikely to replace medical doctors altogether anytime soon unless you are a patient of Medical Officer "Bones" McCoy on *Star Trek*'s USS *Enterprise*, where he could diagnose and cure everything on everybody using a wand.

Medicine's long history encompasses religious dogma, magical thinking, empiricism, and other mindful manipulations. Ancient practitioners would taste urine to see if it attracted ants (to diagnose diabetes) and visually and olfactorily analyzed excrement, hopefully not by tasting it too.

For treatment, doctors used dances, colored lights, readings of crystals or minerals, bloodletting with or without leeches, concoctions of herbs and animal parts such as rhinoceros horns (resulting in the risk of their extinction), and other so-called "natural" therapies.

When MDs and DOs receive evidence-based medicine (EBM) proof that diagnostic and treatment methods used in alternative medicine are effective, they incorporate them into their sound medical practice. Tests and treatments that cannot be proven effective are disregarded. However, they may continue to be found, almost exclusively, in "functional," "complementary," "alternative," and "integrative" health care (CAIH).

Today's medicine is rooted in health science, mathematics and statistical analysis, chemistry and physics, molecular biology, biomedical technology, engineering, public health, psychology, sociology, genetics, immunology, anatomy, tissue histology, pathology, pharmacology, physiology, and physiopathology; these are just some of the pillars of effective clinical practice, rather than being based on gut feelings, assumptions, personal experiences, etc.

Sir Isaac Newton said he made progress by "standing on the shoulders of giants"; medical doctors could say they do it by "standing on the shoulders of other doctors."

Although not just by itself, the current "dogma" in patient care, medical practice, and education is based on the best available evidence of benefit, expert opinions, clinicians' teachings, advancing technologies, and more.

Alternatives to EBM include quackery, a form of health care- or the lack of it- that persists because it is practiced by charlatans and others who feign medical skills; these individuals were described in the preface and identified as quacks.

Medical doctors, myself included, believe that it is the uninformed and desperate patient who is most vulnerable to becoming the prey of those quacks who operate outside of good, proper, and honest medicine.

Although most quackery is found in CAIH, it disappoints me that some bona fide MDs and DOs derail and join the ranks of the quacks. Examples include some homeopaths, functional medicine practitioners, and naturopaths.

I hope what you learn in this book will help you avoid the wrong "practitioners" and "providers."

Who, then, ought to practice medicine?

In the US, medicine is practiced within a healthcare system regulated by both federal and local government agencies. Ultimately, licenses are granted by the state where a provider practices or resides.

Strong regulations limit the scope of practice of legitimate healthcare providers, including MDs and DOs. These regulations feel enforced more strictly for us than for quacks and similar providers. Quacks and other fraudsters somehow circumvent government ordinances. So, follow my advice and learn to be discerning and picky.

In many countries, governments issue credentials that determine who is qualified to practice medicine and, by virtue of their education, is entitled to establish doctor-patient relationships and charge for their services. Those governments also decide who cannot practice and enforce that decision.

In the United States, medical doctors (MDs) receive a comprehensive education at medical schools accredited by the Liaison Committee on Medical Education (LCME), jointly sponsored by the Association of American Medical Colleges (AAMC) and the Council on Medical Education of the American Medical Association (AMA).

Those who are DOs have attended medical schools accredited by the American Osteopathic Association's (AOA) Commission on Osteopathic College Accreditation (COCA). While there are some differences in curricula and accreditation standards, MD and DO schools generally cover the same material.

Another organization, the Educational Council for Foreign Medical Graduates (ECFMG), assesses the readiness of medical doctors who graduated in other countries to enter internships, residencies, or fellowships in accredited US programs (its methodology and relevance are under updating.)

To be granted certification by the ECFMG, graduates must obtain a medical school diploma from an institution registered in the World Directory of Medical Schools and have evidence of successfully completing the United States Medical License Examination (USMLE) Step 1 and Step 2 (and later the Step 3), the same tests taken by American MD graduates.

In US medical schools, candidates to become MDs learn to:

1. Address disease-related complaints by analyzing symptoms, circumstances, history, and epidemiology.
2. Examine for signs or physical findings, interpret information, and reach diagnoses.

3. Explain such diagnoses to patients, relatives, and caretakers.
4. Propose treatment plans, implement them, and follow up on them.

At graduation, MDs are not specialized, and most choose to pursue additional education right away, beginning with internships (considered the first year of residency training) in general or broad fields such as family practice, internal medicine, general surgery, pediatrics, emergency medicine, pathology, or obstetrics and gynecology. Then, they must pass the USMLE Step 3 exam during or after their internship year. Then, they may proceed toward a residency or specialization.

Graduates may continue in these general fields or specialize in areas that include but are not limited to, anesthesia, neurology, psychiatry, physical medicine and rehabilitation, radiology, dermatology, head and neck surgery (otolaryngology), ophthalmology, neurosurgery, orthopedics, urology, and plastic surgery.

Finally, after physicians graduate from their residency training, they may consider further training, which can last from one to three years, in fields such as cardiology, critical care, endocrinology, gastroenterology and hepatology, geriatrics, nephrology, hematology/oncology, infectious disease, immunology and allergy medicine, pulmonology, rheumatology, thoracic (chest) and cardiovascular surgery, trauma surgery, surgical oncology, and colorectal surgery or proctology.

Some specialties, like dermatology, have components that overlap with other fields, including medical, surgical, aesthetic, pediatric, pathological, and immunological. The same could be said of practically every field in medicine. No physician specialty exists in a vacuum.

I bet this is more education than you thought you would get from me. I bet I missed a lot, but I expect you to have gotten the idea: real medical doctors in the United States study long, hard, and a lot.

Throughout their years in practice, generalists and specialists must take many exams to become and stay "board-certified" in ABMS or AOA field members.

Be aware that there are certifying organizations distinct from the ones I just mentioned, some of which you and I should consider suspicious, if not clandestine.

Be aware that the term "board-certified"—like doctor and physician—is being usurped! The ABMS and the AOA websites are good sources of information about recognized specialties and subspecialties (and about their specialists and subspecialists). Legitimate boards are accepted by the most serious medical organizations, including governmental ones, and most countries. As I said above, others may be covert and used by quacks.

What follows illustrates what each medical specialist mostly does without being limited to it:

- Internist or Internal Medicine:

  Diagnosis and treatment of diseases mostly in adult patients.

- Pediatrician:

  Diagnosis and treatment of diseases mostly in children, from neonates to adolescents.

- Geriatrician:

  Diagnosis and treatment of diseases mainly in the elderly, nursing homes, and memory loss patient care.

- Family Practitioner:

  Prevention, triage, well-being, and essential primary care in general. Diagnosis and treatment of common acute and chronic conditions.

- Emergency Physician:

  Diagnosis and treatment of emergent and acute medical conditions are seen in the emergency room (ER) and acute and urgent care.

- Radiologist and Imaging Specialist:

  Interpretation of diagnostic imaging, including X-rays, ultrasound, magnetic resonance (MRI), computerized tomography (CT), and positron emission tomography (PET).

- Allergist and Immunologist:

  Diagnosis and treatment of airway allergies, such as asthma, hay fever, sinusitis; seasonal conjunctivitis; immune disorders; transplant complications; allergic reactions affecting the skin; and more.

- Pathologist:

  Interpret biopsies (tissue analysis), autopsies, laboratory tests, and forensics.

- Obstetrician / Gynecologist:

  Diagnosis and treatment of diseases and conditions affecting women's health, birth control, fertility, pregnancy, vaginal, ovarian and uterine issues, sexually transmitted diseases, and more.

- Psychiatrist:

  Diagnosis and treatment of mental disorders, neurosis, psychosis, depression, anxiety, hallucinations, suicidal ideations, drug dependency, alcoholism, and more.

- Neurologist:

  Diagnosis and treatment of diseases involving the brain, nerves, and muscles, including pain (e.g., headaches), seizures, movement disorders, and memory loss.

- Cardiologist:

  Diagnosis and treatment of heart and blood vessel diseases, failure, medical treatment or stent placement, chest pain, hypertension, leg, ankle, and foot edema, ulcers, and more.

- Nephrologist:

  Diagnosis and treatment of kidney diseases, hypertension, dialysis, renal transplants, and metabolic and electrolytic issues.

- Endocrinologist:

  Diagnosis and treatment of hormonal and metabolic disorders, including eating, obesity, diabetes, thyroid disease, adrenal disease, and more.

- Gastroenterologist:

  Diagnosis and treatment of diseases of the esophagus, stomach, intestines, liver, pancreas, and transplants.

- Pulmonologist:

  Diagnosis and treatment of diseases of the airways and lungs, tuberculosis, fungal and other infections, and lung transplants.

- Rheumatologist:

  Diagnosis and treatment of diseases of the joints, tendons, muscles, and bones, auto-immune disorders (e.g., lupus, scleroderma, and others), and osteo-rheumatoid-psoriatic-arthritis.

- Infectiologist:

  Diagnosis and treatment of infectious diseases, including viral (e.g., HIV/AIDS, COVID-19, and others), bacterial, deep fungal, and parasitic, as well as their complications.

- Hematologist and Oncologist:

  Diagnosis and treatment of anemia, sickle-cell disease, clotting disorders, leukemia and lymphomas, and solid organ (e.g., breasts, lungs, brain, prostate, testicles, colon, and others) cancers.

- Physiatrist:

  Diagnosis and treatment of conditions regarding disability, sports medicine, physical fitness, rehabilitation (stroke, injuries), and pain.

- General Surgeon:

  Diagnosis and treatment of a wide variety of essential surgical procedures, though typically involving the abdomen.

- Trauma Surgeon

  Diagnosis and treatment of acute injuries (accidental and intentional) requiring surgery, as well as management of the surgical intensive care unit.

- Orthopedic Surgeon:

  Diagnosis and treatment of conditions requiring surgery involving the bone, muscle, and joints.

- Head and Neck and Maxillofacial Surgeon:

  Diagnosis and treatment, including surgery, of conditions involving the jaw, mouth, and oral cavity.

- Otolaryngologist:

  Diagnosis and treatment, including surgery, of conditions involving the ear, nose, and throat.

- Ophthalmologist:

  Diagnosis and treatment of conditions affecting the eye, eyelid, orbit surgery, and medicine, including laser, lenses, and other means of vision correction.

- Cardiovascular and Thoracic (Chest) Surgeon:

  Diagnosis and treatment, including surgery, of conditions involving the heart, blood vessels, large and small arteries and veins (including varices), chest wall (ribs vessels, nerves, and muscles in between plus linings), and lung surgery.

- Neurosurgeon:

  Diagnosis and treatment, including surgery, of conditions involving the brain, such as brain tumors or cancer, stroke, spine (deformities, tumors), peripheral nerve repair, and pain (relating to the back).

- Surgical Oncologist:

  Diagnosis and treatment, including surgery, of cancers. They can be general or specialized.

- Colon and Rectum Surgeon / Proctologist:

  Diagnosis and treatment, including surgery, of conditions involving the anus, rectum, and colon, such as bleeding fissures, hemorrhoids, warts, tumors, cancer, and inflammation.

- Urologist:

  Diagnosis and treatment, including surgery, of conditions involving the penis, kidneys, and urine pathways (ureters, bladder, urethra), such as stones, infections, and tumors.

- Plastic Surgeon:

  Reconstructive and cosmetic surgeries and procedures throughout the body. Surgical management of injuries and conditions involving the hand.

- Dermatologist:

  Diagnosis and treatment of diseases involving the skin, hair, and nails. Dermatologic surgery, cryosurgery, and cosmetic procedures.

- Anesthesiologist:

  Pre-operative sedation, pain avoidance, and pain medicine.

- Preventive and Aerospace Medicine specialist:

  Epidemiology and public health prevention and control, occupational medicine, and aerospace disease avoidance and treatment.

- Nuclear Medicine Specialist:

  Diagnosis and therapy utilizing atomic and sub-atomic particles, mainly of cancer.

- Medical Geneticist:

  Diagnosis and evaluations of genetic and inheritable disorders and development of treatments.

I am appalled that, as daunting and complex as the education and training of doctors in the preceding list of generalists and specialists is, some real MDs and DOs deviate towards practice forms of health care that are considered different from the kind they went to school to learn. Fortunately, this happens rarely.

As an MD friend would have said, "God bless them." (I'm not sure if he was being sarcastic.)

As you have probably noticed, I wrote this guide to expose healthcare professionals who, not being educated in medical schools that train MDs or DOs, attempt to infringe upon the legitimate field of medicine, masquerade as "doctors," and to safeguard patients from them.

To reduce confusion and to organize and simplify readers' thoughts, I created the following list of healthcare professionals who are not MDs or DOs:

- Eye Doctor (Optometrist) (OD)
- Foot Doctor (Podiatrist) (DPM)
- Doctor of Chiropractic (Chiropractor, DC)
- Audiologist (AuD, Hearing Doctor)
- Psychologist, Psychotherapist, Psychoanalyst (PsyD)
- Physician Assistant (PA)
- Naturopathic Physician (ND, NMD)
- Functional Medicine Practitioner (FMP)
- Complementary, Alternative, and Integrative Health (CAIH)
- Nutritionist / Nutriologist
- Registered Dietitian (RD)
- Nurse Practitioner (NP)
- Nurse Injector (typically a registered nurse [RN] or NP)
- Certified Registered Nurse Anesthetist (CRNA)
- Certified Nurse Midwife (CNM)
- Physical Therapist (PT, DPT)
- Dental Assistant, Dental Therapist

The preceding list does not imply that those professionals do not play an invaluable role in patient care; most do, especially when part of a team supervised by MDs or DOs. Instead, it is intended to clarify who does not go through medical or osteopathic school so you can catch them if they portray themselves as doctors of medicine before they cause harm.

References and Recommended Reading

1. "Quackwatch," Center for Inquiry, https://quackwatch.org.
2. "American Osteopathic Association," American Osteopathic Association, http://www.osteopathic.org/inside-aoa/development/aoa-board-certification/Pages/specialty-subspecialty-certification.aspx.
3. *Skeptic Magazine*, www.skeptic.com.
4. Committee for Skeptical Inquiry, www.csicop.org.
5. American Board of Medical Specialties, www.abms.org.
6. Federation of State Medical Boards, https://www.fsmb.org.
7. Educational Commission for Foreign Medical Graduates, http://www.ecfmg.org.
8. United States Medical Licensing Examination, http://www.usmle.org.

What Is Evidence-Based Medicine (EBM)?

Evidence-based medicine (EBM) is regarded as the most appropriate and essential approach to practicing medicine, teaching it, and delivering good health care.

EBM results from careful, deliberate, and explicit use of up-to-date information obtained from valid, relevant, and systematic research using the scientific method, which is then integrated into clinical practice.

EBM advocates that decisions regarding a patient's medical care should primarily be supported by evidence of effectiveness, rated on a scale from nil to weak to strong, rather than by the beliefs of experts and practitioners. It also identifies harmful treatments and practices, eliminating them from clinical practice.

Using EBM removes subjectivity from clinical judgment, reducing bias influenced by a doctor's beliefs. As a result, patient care becomes more precise. It necessitates systematic reviews of published medical research to significantly influence how diagnostic and therapeutic paths are chosen.

However, EBM can be time-consuming, difficult to implement, impractical, and sometimes unattainable for practicing physicians. It requires reviewing and scrutinizing large volumes of medical literature related to each patient's diagnosis and treatment needs. Despite these challenges, medical certifying bodies have made continuing medical education (education that occurs after graduation and licensure) mandatory to ensure that physicians stay current.

Fortunately, professional organizations exist that are equipped to systematically review, organize, examine, appraise, and synthesize vast quantities of high-quality medical information for physicians who require them. AI is poised to enhance and expedite much of that search effort and may soon serve as a platform for accurate, quality medical practice.

An excellent and important example of an organization that effectively processes medical information is the Cochrane Collaboration, a global, independent, not-for-profit network comprising healthcare practitioners, researchers, patient advocates, and others dedicated to generating credible and accessible medical information for free, independent of commercial sponsorship and potential conflicts of interest. The Cochrane Collaboration is highly regarded as a reliable source of practical medical knowledge, which I find extremely helpful in my everyday practice and in teaching my resident physicians.

EBM is now taught at all medical schools and practiced by all competent doctors. I am confident you will guess and understand why I recommend choosing physicians who use EBM. Patients should feel free to ask their doctors whether they use it and to provide documentation proving so, taking time to explain the diagnosis, how treatments work, success rates, frequency of adverse effects, and so on. And you thought Bugs Bunny was being funny; we now recognize how clever he was whenever he asked, "What's up, Doc?"

The answer to "Are you basing my diagnosis and treatment on EBM?" could effectively eliminate functional and other

CAIH practitioners and quacks unless they lie to your face, as they likely do not use it. However, since quacks are quite clever, they may still attempt to find ways to deceive you, so remain cautious and inquisitive.

While browsing books on hypnosis, I noticed some that claimed to be "evidence-based." However, as I flipped through their pages, it became clear that they were misusing the term, presumably for marketing advantage.

Eliminating them from the picture will help lessen the risk of harm and simplify decisions on whom to consult for medical attention.

References and Recommended Reading

1. David L. Sackett, William M. C. Rosenberg, J. A. Muir Gray, R. Brian Haynes, W. Scott Richardson, "Evidence-Based Medicine: What It Is and What It Isn't," *British Medical Journal*, 1996; 312(7023): 71–72, https://doi.org/10.1136/bmj.312.7023.71.
2. Cochrane.org, www.cochrane.org.

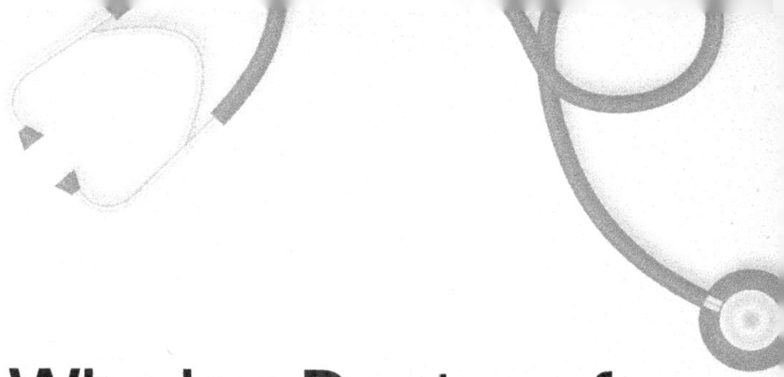

Who Is a Doctor of Medicine (MD)?

Medical doctors (MDs) are the quintessential experts in diagnosis, treatment, and patient care.

They achieve this through rigorous higher education in disease prevention, diagnosis, and treatment training. Their goal is to cure patients when possible and offer relief when it is not.

MDs are expected to diagnose, treat, explain diseases, and develop care plans using information based on facts, scientific knowledge, and experience.

They offer the highest levels of care in health and disease, being the most in-depth and in-extension-trained professionals, the "gold standard," so to speak, in the medical field.

MDs are understandably protective of their turf, which is constantly probed by a variety of mid-educated, less competent, and less prepared providers seeking to invade it for two main reasons:

1. They zealously care for the well-being of patients.
2. They underwent the most extensive and rigorous education process in the field of medicine. Therefore, they consider it inappropriate and unacceptable that less-trained providers, such as MEPs or quacks, pretend

to compete with them without making an equivalent effort.

The career for an MD starts off being quite demanding and never ends being so.

MDs practice less for the money (as I hear some people say or read in their minds) and more for many other gratifications, like the great feeling of curing somebody.

Typically, an MD's education requires four years of undergraduate studies in pre-medicine fields, which must be completed with an average grade point average (GPA) of at least 3.8 and, more likely 4.0.

Before applying to medical school, applicants must take the Medical College Admission Test (MCAT). This exam evaluates problem-solving skills, critical reading, critical thinking, and understanding of natural, behavioral, and social science concepts and principles, which are essential prerequisites for studying and ultimately practicing medicine.

The MCAT, administered by the Association of American Medical Colleges (AAMC), is challenging to score well on. It is a significant filter for pre-medical students entering medical school. Currently, acceptable students are expected to be in the top quartile of MCAT scores.

Four more years are then to be spent in medical school.

In the first two years, medical students learn about physiology, biomechanics, anatomy, histology and cytology, pathology, biochemistry, genetics, microbiology, immunology, pharmacology, toxicology, epidemiology, public health, statistics, nutrition, neuroscience, and a lot more.

In the next two years (the clinical education phase), medical students learn to diagnose medical conditions or diseases and develop appropriate treatment plans. This is accomplished through hands-on rotations in internal medicine, surgery, pediatrics, psychiatry, obstetrics and gynecology, and other departments and various other specialties. During these rotations, medical students work directly with and under resident and attending physicians to develop and enhance their clinical interviewing and physical examination skills. They then propose and receive feedback on their diagnosis and care plan.

Alongside regularly attending various formal lectures by experts in specific medical fields—often more than once a day—and spending nights caring for patients, medical students participate in rounds with faculty professors, ideally to learn from the best and most experienced.

At the end of these four years, the MD degree may be conferred upon those who pass all phases of the medical school training tests and obtain recommendations from the faculty who instructed them.

Then, another significant stumbling block or filter arises: an organization known as the United States Medical Licensing Examination (USMLE), sponsored by the Federation of State Medical Boards (FSMB) and the National Board of Medical Examiners (NBME). This organization assesses a medical student's ability, as a future physician, to apply the knowledge, principles, and concepts acquired in medical school and to demonstrate the essential patient-centered skills that are critical in health and disease, forming the foundation for safe and effective patient care. The examinations conducted by the USMLE have three components called "Steps."

To take the first two Steps, an applicant must be enrolled in or have graduated from a US or Canadian medical school, which leads to obtaining the MD or DO degree.

After the first two years of medical school, students take Step 1. This exam evaluates their understanding and ability to apply key concepts from the basic sciences to medical practice, focusing on the principles and mechanisms behind health, disease, and therapy. Up to 280 questions are presented over a period of eight hours.

After the third year of medical school, students take Step 2, which assesses their ability to apply medical knowledge, skills, and understanding of clinical science essential for providing patient care across all specialties. It emphasizes health promotion and disease prevention, with approximately 318 questions to be answered over nine hours.

During or after completing an internship year of residency, an MD can sit for the Step 3 exam. This assessment measures the ability to apply medical knowledge and understanding of biomedical or clinical science essential for the unsupervised practice of medicine. It is conducted over two days, with the first day lasting seven hours and the second lasting over nine hours. In total, about 412 questions are asked, and thirteen computer-based simulations must be completed.

To take Step 3, a DO must have already obtained a DO degree from a medical school accredited by the Liaison Committee on Medical Education (LCME) or the American Osteopathic Association (AOA) in the US or Canada. While DOs do not need to take Step 3 and may choose to complete the COMLEX Level 3 instead, many DOs aiming for medical fellowships after residency training opt to take Step 3.

In most states, to be licensed to practice medicine without supervision, a year of internship is added to passing all three USMLE Steps for an MD or the three COMLEX Levels for DOs.

As this issue concerns some members of our society, I'll dedicate the next few lines to the situation of foreign medical graduates (FMGs). Some may have received training that did not meet the standards set by the GPAs or MCATs of US candidates, prompting them to attend schools abroad or study medicine in other countries. However, to enter American residency programs, FMGs must demonstrate that their qualifications meet the requirements of the Educational Council for Foreign Medical Graduates (ECFMG). They must also take an English exam to prove their fluency. Once approved, they can proceed with their postgraduate medical education in the US. FMGs must take the USMLE Step exams, not the COMLEX Level exams, and typically, they must score in the top quartile.

After graduation and a year of internship, the residency process begins; this can take another two to six years. Upon successful completion of residency, MDs (and DOs) qualify to take another test, the board certification in the specialty in which they complete their residency.

As you may have noticed by now, the MD or DO has spent approximately eleven to fifteen years, or more, obtaining the medical education that patients expect and value.

But there's more! MDs can pursue fellowships, typically in a subspecialty or different specialty, adding another three years to their education. Consequently, the total duration of their higher education becomes twelve to eighteen years.

MDs can choose to enter a general field, such as family practice, internal medicine, or surgery, and later select a specialty, like rheumatology or surgical oncology, or a subspecialty, such as pediatric cardiology. For nearly all specialties, an MD must first complete an internship year. After finishing a residency in a specialty, the MD may qualify for yet another challenge: the board certification test.

Keep in mind that interns and residents typically work intensely for over sixty hours a week, sometimes even eighty or more. In contrast, many other medical professions require only thirty-six to forty hours per week. Additionally, many residents do not have weekends or holidays off. A few decades ago, during my training, we often worked upwards of one hundred hours a week, with every third night on call. This could summarize my weekly schedule in hours: 24 + 12 + 12 + 24 + 12 + 12 + 24 = 120. Of course, not every week began and ended with twenty-four-hour days, so some weeks were 'only' 108 hours long at the hospital. Mathematically speaking, this number of hours and their intensity doubles the time that MDs and DOs spend compared to other healthcare providers. In other words, the three to seven years of training effectively compares to nine to fifteen years, as the time MDs spend in internship, residency, and fellowship greatly exceeds that of most pretenders.

Beyond that, medical education never finishes.

Board certifications typically remain valid for ten years, depending on the specialty. The preparation for renewal processes and tests is rigorous and complicated, demanding significant effort and personal sacrifice.

In addition, MDs continue studying independently, including before and after each challenging patient encounter, attending hospital-based conferences that may happen weekly, if not daily, or medical meetings and conventions to keep up with the latest information and trade knowledge amongst colleagues.

I hope that the information provided above has helped you gain respect for the doctoral degrees earned by MDs and DOs and has clarified why they are so protective of their field against intruders with significantly less training.

Many MDs, like DOs, dislike being called providers because this equates them with mid-medically educated practitioners (MEPs) and other intruders into the medical field, including quacks).

References and Recommended Reading

1. "Occupational Outlook Handbook: Physicians and Surgeons," Bureau of Labor Statistics, US Department of Labor, https://www.bls.gov/ooh/healthcare/physicians-and-surgeons.htm.
2. "Home | United States Medical Licensing Examination," United States Medical Licensing Examination, www.usmle.org/.

Who Is a Doctor of Osteopathy (DO)?

The only physicians, aside from MDs, licensed to practice medicine independently in the US are doctors of osteopathic medicine (DOs).

While the osteopathic approach to healthcare differs somewhat from traditional methods, laws in all U.S. states recognize DO and MD degrees as equivalent. I'd like to share a brief story to illustrate the differences in their philosophies.

The history of osteopathy began with Andrew Taylor Still, an MD who, discontented with the ineffectiveness of nineteenth-century medicine, pioneered osteopathic medicine in 1874. He believed that the musculoskeletal system was an essential part of health and that medical care could be enhanced through the use of manual techniques alongside medication. He established the first osteopathic school in Missouri in 1892. Today, there are nearly 150,000 to 200,000 DOs, and the number of schools offering osteopathy and its registrants is growing rapidly. I would like to see a similar impetus from the MD side in the hope of training more fully educated physicians in lieu of the mid-educated providers.

Traditionally, osteopathic medicine asserts that the body is "more capable of self-regulation and healing as a unit that combines body, mind, and spirit." Consequently, some view the addition of osteopathic manipulative therapy (OMT), a hands-on manipulation practiced to correct somatic dysfunctions, as therapeutic.

In OMT, joints and muscles are moved, resisted, and stretched to correct somatic dysfunctions, which aim to fix structural imbalances, improve circulation, and relieve pain.

DOs, like MDs, complete higher education and rigorous residency training to learn how to prevent, diagnose, and treat diseases. They earn their degrees at osteopathic schools, which nowadays offer curriculums similar to those of MD schools. Most DOs train under MD attendings alongside MD students and residents during clinical rotations and as residents.

DOs recommend a holistic (considering the patient as a whole—shouldn't that then be a "wholistic" or "wholeistic"?) approach to treatment rather than focusing on a specific diseased body part, organ, or system. They are, or used to be, prescribers of medications only when deemed necessary.

I'm concerned that the concept of "holistic" has been hijacked by DOs; worse still, by CAIH practitioners like chiropractors and naturopaths, which I believe is for marketing purposes that extend beyond what may benefit patients.

Similar to DOs, MDs do not see a malfunctioning organ as separate from the individual it belongs to. MDs do not treat livers; instead, they treat individuals with liver disease. In that regard, all MDs practice holistically.

Another difference between DOs and MDs relates to accessibility.

The current ratio of practicing DOs to MDs is approximately one to four or five, with around 150,000 to 200,000 DOs and about 900,000 MDs. However, this gap is narrowing.

Candidates who enter osteopathic school typically complete four years of undergraduate studies, graduating with an average GPA of over 3.6 (versus closer to 3.8 to 4.0 for MD schools). This difference is significant in statistical terms.

Like MD candidates, DO candidates start building their résumés with experiences as young as high school.

The rigors of the MCAT also filter out osteopathic candidates. Their average score is 504, the 62nd percentile, compared to 512 for MD candidates, which is the 83rd percentile. Higher acceptance rates into osteopathic (versus MD) schools hint at less stringent requirements.

Medical school curricula for DOs and MDs are similarly structured. They offer two years of basic knowledge and two years of hands-on clinical rotations.

Unlike MDs, DOs are not required to take Step 1 at the end of the first two years, yet about half do, mostly to get into the more competitive residency programs.

Instead of the Step exams, DOs take the Comprehensive Osteopathic Medical Licensure Examination (COMLEX), which resembles the USMLE that MD students take. COMLEX Level 1 is a nine-hour exam with 352 questions that test foundational medical sciences, such as body systems physiology, anatomy, pharmacology, and pathology, and adds OMT.

After their third year of medical school, DO students take the COMLEX Level 2CK test, another nine-hour exam with 400 questions. Some also opt to take Step 2 of the USMLE, again hoping to broaden their residency options.

DOs take COMLEX Level 3 during or after their intern year, whereas MDs take USMLE Step 3. The COMLEX Level 3 is a two-day examination of 420 questions and twenty-six clinical decision-making (CDM) cases.

During schooling, DOs study about 300 to 500 additional hours of training in OMT compared to MDs to obtain their degree, something they often later drop from practice. Some say this is because OMT is not reimbursed well, considering the time required. Others may not agree with the purported therapeutic benefits of OMT.

Again, the most notable differences between DOs and MDs are philosophical and relatively minor.

The COMLEX and USMLE tests differ because their results are not comparable. Therefore, the public can only use the COMLEX website's percentile calculator to deduce whether one group of students is better prepared.

After graduation, DOs can enroll in residency programs just like MDs. Some DOs choose and may be accepted into MD residencies, while others stay in primarily DO programs.

In 2020, the AOA (DO) and ACGME (MD) residency accrediting bodies merged. AOA programs that met ACGME requirements became incorporated, and those that didn't should have been disbanded.

Under this new system, all residents (DO or MD) in ACGME programs meet similar, rigorous training requirements and take the same set of in-training examinations.

Like MDs, DOs train for at least three years in residency for specialties like family medicine and emergency medicine and five to seven years for general surgery and neurosurgery. Some go on to subspecialize in their designated fields, leading to another one to three years of training.

DOs, like MDs, spend nine to fifteen years in internships, residencies, and fellowships. They update and enhance their medical knowledge with continuous medical education (CME) programs and renew their license by taking maintenance board exams every ten years.

Having taught and currently teaching in postgraduate programs that admit DOs and MDs, I can attest that the quality of healthcare delivered by DOs is comparable to that of MDs. If there is any difference, it varies from one resident to another. However, the public still perceives this difference to favor MDs.

It doesn't help DOs' reputation that some engage in dubious practices like chelation, "cranial therapy," and "visceral manipulation."

Unlike MD degrees, DO degrees are not universally recognized. In many countries, DOs cannot prescribe medications, and their status as equals to MDs is not embraced. In the US, some phone directories still list DOs separately from MDs.

Based on US policies and my experiences as a medical educator, I consider DOs to be equally competent as MDs in providing quality healthcare, particularly those DOs who have been recently trained. However, like many MDs, I find OMT unnecessary.

References and Recommended Reading

1. American Osteopathic Association, https://osteopathic.org.
2. American Osteopathic Association. Osteopathic Medical Profession Report. Chicago, IL, http://www.osteopathic.org/inside-aoa/about/who-we-are/Documents/Osteopathic-Medical-Profession-Report-2010.pdf.
3. Stephen Barrett, "Dubious Aspects of Osteopathy," Quackwatch, February 11, 2018, http://quackwatch.com/04Consumer Education/QA/osteo.html.
4. Stephen Salzberg, "Osteopathic Physicians versus Doctors," *Forbes*, October 27, 2010, https://www.forbes.com/sites/sciencebiz/2010/10/27/osteopaths-versus-doctors/.

What Is the American Board of Medical Specialties (ABMS)?

Some MDs, DOs, and non-physician providers (NPPs) claim board certifications. However, the certifications—particularly those of the latter—often come from dubious or questionable organizations, which prevents the public from viewing them as fraudulent.

I wrote this chapter, along with a couple of others, to clarify what is accurate and meaningful regarding board certifications and what is not.

In another chapter, I share a story about an incident at my office that highlights the misuse of titles by NPPs. A PA claimed she was "board-certified in dermatology" when all she had completed was a weekend course. She presented a diploma that merely confirmed her attendance as proof. She used it to mislead our appointment clerk. These days, anyone can create a fake diploma, so it's wise to be suspicious. (caveat emptor.)

A dermatologist like me must complete a three-year residency program (after internship) to qualify for and pass the board test sanctioned by the American Board of Dermatology (ABD). A family practitioner who states, "Practice limited to dermatology," cannot be certified by the ABD. Only those who have spent three years in an accredited dermatology residency program can pursue that certification. I mention this field because I am knowledgeable about it; other specialists can express similar discontent when they see their board certification usurped.

Although the language I use from here on may not be as clear as I would prefer, I utilize it because I need to paraphrase legal content that belongs to specific organizations and was likely drafted by their attorneys. My apologies, but you all understand how lawyers communicate using a lingo often difficult to grasp, self-serving, and laden with complicated jargon. Capish?

The American Board of Medical Specialties (ABMS) is an organization of twenty-four member medical specialties that defines the qualifications for many specialties and provides the examinations MDs and DOs must take to become board-certified.

Board certifications are voluntary for physicians and are not required to practice. However, a specific institution or medical organization, such as a hospital or academic program, may require them to conduct research. Boards may also become necessary to maintain state licensure, something I find abusive and inappropriate. Still, I keep up with mine.

A certification from the appropriate board should reassure the public that a specific physician is an expert in their field and stays current. The ABMS oversees board certifications in many specialties, believing that the higher standards physicians must meet will improve patient outcomes and care.

As discussed in earlier chapters, MDs and some DOs must complete a rigorous process to become board-certified. After extensive training in an accredited residency program, they must pass both written and occasionally oral exams administered by a specialty board member of the ABMS.

To maintain board certification, physicians must go through a process formerly known as Maintenance of Certification (MOC), which is now called the Continuance of Certification Program (CCP). This process consists of a series of steps that culminate in re-certifying exams, administered every ten years or adapted as an ongoing assessment designed to demonstrate that a physician possesses current expertise in a specialty, commitment to patient care, and proficiency in communication and ethics.

The ABMS offers a Certification Verification Service that lets the public check if a physician is truly board-certified in a given specialty.

A small number of doctors and many imposters falsely claim to be board-certified when they are not, at least not by a board recognized by the ABMS or AOA.

Identifying individuals who are not certified but claim to be is essential. Their practices can be misleading, which is unethical, and we want to avoid that. With this in mind, I invite you to read the ABPS chapter.

For example, plastic surgeons who perform beautifying procedures like facelifts and breast augmentations, repair faces after car accidents, reconstruct and replace physical defects, perform hand surgery, and manage burn care are only recognized by the ABMS through the American Board of Plastic Surgery, not by other boards labeled as "cosmetic," "aesthetic," or "facial plastic." The absence of board certification from an ABMS-recognized or AOA-recognized board does not indicate a lack of competence; it simply means that the stringent requirements of a member specialty board were not fulfilled.

"Plastic surgeons" who do not qualify for certification from the American Board of Plastic Surgery (ABPS) or who have not taken or passed its exam may claim certification from other "boards" with names that might be fabricated, such as the "Board of Facial Plastic" or "Cosmetic Surgery." These board certifications may be provided by organizations other than the ABPS, including the questionable (to me and many colleagues) American Board of Physician Specialties (ABPS).

The idea behind claiming such contrived certifications is likely to market services or deceive patients. I often see those advertisements in phonebooks, newspapers, car wash magazines, and electronic media. Caveat emptor!

A cornucopia of academies, associations, societies, and other catchy names for medical aggrupations—welcoming, legally representing, and providing credentials similar to board certifications for physicians and other providers—has developed recently. I would stick to the boards recognized by the ABMS for MDs and the AOA for DOs. Caveat emptor!

Next, I will provide a list of the medical specialties and subspecialties recognized by the ABMS. You are encouraged to use this list to verify whether your medical doctor is certified in one or more of these areas. If you have any doubts, utilize the verification systems they offer.

American Board of Allergy and Immunology

- Allergy and Immunology
- No subspecialties

American Board of Anesthesiology

- Anesthesiology
- Critical Care Medicine
- Neurocritical Care

- Hospice and Palliative Medicine
- Pain Medicine
- Sleep Medicine
- Pediatric Anesthesiology
- Adult Cardiac Anesthesiology

American Board of Colon and Rectal Surgery

- Colon and Rectal Surgery
- No subspecialties

American Board of Dermatology

- Dermatology
- Dermatopathology
- Pediatric Dermatology
- Micrographic Dermatologic Surgery

American Board of Emergency Medicine

- Emergency Medicine
- Anesthesiology Critical Care Medicine
- Emergency Medical Services
- Hospice and Palliative Medicine
- Internal Medicine-Critical Care Medicine
- Medical Toxicology
- Neurocritical Care
- Pain Medicine
- Pediatric Emergency Medicine
- Pediatric Emergency Medicine
- Sports Medicine
- Undersea and Hyperbaric Medicine

American Board of Family Medicine

- Family Medicine
- Adolescent Medicine
- Geriatric Medicine
- Hospice and Palliative Medicine
- Pain Medicine
- Sleep Medicine
- Sports Medicine

American Board of Internal Medicine

- Internal Medicine
- Adolescent Medicine
- Adult Congenital Heart Disease
- Advanced Heart Failure and Transplant Cardiology
- Cardiovascular Disease
- Clinical Cardiac Electrophysiology
- Critical Care Medicine
- Endocrinology, Diabetes, and Metabolism
- Gastroenterology
- Geriatric Medicine
- Hematology
- Hospice and Palliative Medicine
- Infectious Disease
- Interventional Cardiology
- Medical Oncology
- Nephrology
- Neurocritical Care
- Pulmonary Disease
- Rheumatology
- Sleep Medicine
- Sports Medicine

- Transplant Hepatology

American Board of Medical Genetics and Genomics

- Clinical Biochemical Genetics
- Clinical Genetics and Genomics (MD)
- Laboratory Genetics and Genomics
- Medical Biochemical Genetics
- Medical Genetic Pathology

American Board of Neurological Surgery

- Neurological Surgery
- Neurocritical Care

American Board of Nuclear Medicine

- Nuclear Medicine
- No subspecialties

American Board of Obstetrics and Gynecology

- Obstetrics and Gynecology
- Complex Family Planning
- Critical Care Medicine
- Female Pelvic Medicine and Reconstructive Surgery
- Gynecologic Oncology
- Maternal-Fetal Medicine
- Reproductive Endocrinology and Infertility

American Board of Ophthalmology

- Ophthalmology
- No subspecialties

American Board of Orthopedic Surgery

- Orthopedic Surgery
- Orthopedic Sports Medicine
- Surgery of the Hand

American Board of Otolaryngology-Head and Neck Surgery

- Otolaryngology-Head and Neck Surgery
- Complex Pediatric Otolaryngology
- Neurotology
- Plastic Surgery within the Head and Neck
- Sleep Medicine

American Board of Pathology

- Pathology—Anatomic/Pathology—Clinical
- Pathology—Anatomic
- Pathology—Clinical
- Blood Banking / Transfusion Medicine
- Clinical Informatics
- Cytopathology
- Dermatopathology
- Hematopathology
- Neuropathology
- Pathology—Chemical
- Pathology—Forensic
- Pathology—Medical Microbiology
- Pathology—Molecular Genetic
- Pathology—Pediatric

American Board of Pediatrics

- Pediatrics
- Adolescent Medicine

- Child Abuse Pediatrics
- Developmental-Behavioral Pediatrics
- Hospice and Palliative Medicine
- Medical Toxicology
- Neonatal-Perinatal Medicine
- Pediatric Cardiology
- Pediatric Critical Care Medicine
- Pediatric Emergency Medicine
- Pediatric Endocrinology
- Pediatric Gastroenterology
- Pediatric Hematology-Oncology
- Pediatric Hospital Medicine
- Pediatric Infectious Diseases
- Pediatric Nephrology
- Pediatric Pulmonology
- Pediatric Rheumatology
- Pediatric Transplant Hepatology
- Sleep Medicine
- Sports Medicine

American Board of Physical Medicine and Rehabilitation

- Physical Medicine and Rehabilitation
- Brain Injury Medicine
- Neuromuscular Medicine
- Pain Medicine
- Pediatric Rehabilitation Medicine
- Spinal Cord Injury Medicine
- Sports Medicine

American Board of Plastic Surgery

- Plastic Surgery
- Plastic Surgery within the Head and Neck

- Surgery of the Hand

American Board of Preventive Medicine

- Public Health and General Preventive Medicine
- Aerospace Medicine
- Addiction Medicine
- Occupational Medicine
- Clinical Informatics
- Medical Toxicology
- Undersea and Hyperbaric Medicine

American Board of Psychiatry and Neurology

- Psychiatry
- Neurology
- Neurology with Special Qualification in Child Neurology
- Addiction Psychiatry
- Brain Injury Medicine
- Child and Adolescent Psychiatry
- Clinical Neurophysiology
- Consultation-Liaison Psychiatry
- Epilepsy
- Forensic Psychiatry
- Geriatric Psychiatry
- Neurocritical Care
- Neurodevelopmental Disabilities
- Pain Medicine
- Sleep Medicine
- Vascular Neurology

American Board of Radiology

- Diagnostic Radiology

- Interventional Radiology and Diagnostic Radiology
- Medical Physics (Diagnostic, Nuclear, Therapeutic)
- Neuroradiology
- Nuclear Radiology
- Pain Medicine
- Pediatric Radiology
- Radiation Oncology

American Board of Surgery

- General Surgery
- Vascular Surgery
- Complex General Surgical Oncology
- Pediatric Surgery
- Surgery of the Hand
- Surgical Critical Care

American Board of Thoracic Surgery

- Thoracic and Cardiac Surgery
- Congenital Cardiac Surgery

American Board of Urology

- Urology
- Female Pelvic Medicine and Reconstructive Surgery
- Pediatric Urology

The AMA recognizes all ABMS (and AOA) member specialty boards and keeps records of professional education, specialty board certifications, and disciplinary actions.

If your medical doctor claims to be certified in a specialty not recognized by the ABMS, be cautious. Verify with the State Medical Society or State Board where he or she practices to ensure everything is legitimate. Ask him or her why the board he or she professes to belong to does not show his or her name in the listing they or she professes to belong to, ensuring it is in a member board within those above.

References and Recommended Reading

1. American Board of Medical Specialties (ABMS), https://www.abms.org.
2. "Verify Certification," American Board of Medical Specialties, http://www.abms.org/verify-certification/.
3. "Residency Training Requirements for Plastic Surgery," The American Board of Plastic Surgery, Inc., https://www.abplasticsurgery.org/residents/training-requirements/.

What Is the American Osteopathic Association (AOA)?

The American Osteopathic Association (AOA) serves as the main advocacy and accreditation body for osteopathic physicians. It oversees osteopathic medical schools, physician board certification, and advocacy initiatives.

The AOA's Department of Certifying Boards is somewhat equivalent to the ABMS for MDs; in other words, it is the organization that oversees the specialty certifying boards for DOs.

After graduating from an accredited osteopathic school, DOs may opt to become certified by a specialty board recognized by the AOA.

Many DOs choose to become certified by an ABMS specialty board. To do so, they must complete a residency program designed and approved for MDs. Interestingly, MDs were not allowed into residency programs intended for DOs until 2020, when the Accreditation Council for Graduate Medical Education (ACGME) consolidated both fields. In the residency program I oversee, we accept MDs and DOs equally. Still, most MDs prefer to remain on the MD track and not transition to DO residency programs.

Similarly, although not identically to how the ABMS recognizes only certain specialties, the AOA currently approves board certifications in the following specialties and subspecialties:

Anesthesiology

- Anesthesiology
- Critical Care
- Pain Management
- Pediatric Anesthesiology

Dermatology

- Dermatology
- Dermatopathology
- Mohs Micrographic Surgery
- Pediatric Dermatology

Emergency Medicine

- Emergency Medicine
- Emergency Medical Services
- Hospice and Palliative Medicine
- Sports Medicine
- Undersea and Hyperbaric Medicine

Family Physician

- Family Medicine / OMT
- Cranial Osteopathic Manipulation (CAQ)
- Geriatric Medicine
- Addiction Medicine
- Correctional Medicine
- Hospice and Palliative Care Medicine
- Pain Medicine

- Sleep Medicine
- Sports Medicine
- Undersea and Hyperbaric Medicine

Internal Medicine

- Internal Medicine
- Cardiology
- Clinical Cardiac Electrophysiology
- Critical Care Medicine
- Endocrinology
- Gastroenterology
- Geriatric Medicine
- Hematology
- Infectious Disease
- Interventional Cardiology
- Nephrology
- Oncology
- Pulmonary Disease
- Rheumatology
- Addiction Medicine
- Pediatric and Adult Allergy and Immunology
- Correctional Medicine
- Hospice and Palliative Care Medicine
- Pain Medicine
- Sleep Medicine
- Sports Medicine

Neurology and Psychiatry

- Neurology
- Psychiatry
- Child and Adolescent Neurology
- Child and Adolescent Psychiatry

- Geriatric Psychiatry
- Neurophysiology
- Addiction Medicine
- Hospice and Palliative Medicine
- Sleep Medicine

Neuromusculoskeletal Medicine

- Neuromusculoskeletal Medicine and OMM
- No subspecialties

Nuclear Medicine

- Nuclear Medicine
- No subspecialties

Obstetrics and Gynecology

- Obstetrics and Gynecology
- Female Pelvic Medicine and Reconstructive Surgery
- Gynecologic Oncology
- Maternal and Fetal Medicine

Ophthalmology and Otolaryngology-Head and Neck Surgery

- Ophthalmology
- Otolaryngology and Facial Plastic Surgery
- Otolaryngic Allergy
- Sleep Medicine

Orthopedic Surgery

- Orthopedic Surgery
- Hand Surgery
- Orthopedic Sports Medicine

Pathology

- Anatomic Pathology
- Clinical Pathology / Laboratory Medicine
- Forensic Pathology
- Dermatopathology

Pediatrics

- Pediatrics
- Neonatology
- Pediatric and Adult Allergy and Immunology
- Sports Medicine

Physical Medicine and Rehabilitation

- Physical Medicine and Rehabilitation
- Hospice and Palliative Medicine
- Pain Medicine
- Sports Medicine

Preventive Medicine

- Aerospace Medicine
- Occupational and Environmental Medicine
- Public Health and Community Medicine
- Occupational Medicine
- Undersea and Hyperbaric Medicine
- Correctional Medicine

Proctology

- Proctology
- No subspecialties

Radiology

- Diagnostic Radiology
- Radiation Oncology
- Neuroradiology
- Pediatric Radiology
- Vascular and Interventional Radiology

Surgery

- Cardiothoracic Surgery
- General Surgery
- Neurological Surgery
- Plastic and Reconstructive Surgery
- Vascular Surgery
- Urological Surgery
- Surgical Critical Care

Any reader with time to spare will notice that the specialties certified by the AOA and those certified by the ABMS share a lot of similarities.

Confusion can arise between the two groups of doctors because some subspecialties are associated with multiple specialties. For instance, a DO or MD can become a hand surgeon through either plastic or orthopedic surgery, as recognized by the ABMS and the AOA.

When I included both listings in the text, I aimed to offer practical guidance for readers seeking a specialist or subspecialist in either field while simplifying the process of determining whether a particular DO or MD genuinely belongs to a specialty accredited by the AOA or the ABMS, thereby eliminating imposters.

Instead of the tests that MDs use to maintain their certification, DOs are required to complete at least 120 hours of continuing medical education every three years and successfully demonstrate their maintenance of specialty skills and knowledge necessary for the correct practice of osteopathy. The AOA recently added a process for continuous recertification, the osteopathic continuous certification.

The ABMS and the AOA should continue collaborating to clearly define which specialties and subspecialties are included in their memberships. This can help the public understand the perceived differences between MDs and DOs.

References and Recommended Reading

1. "AOA Board Certification," American Osteopathic Association, http://www.osteopathic.org/inside-aoa/development/aoa-board-certification/Pages/default.aspx.
2. "Osteopathic Continuous Certification," American Osteopathic Association, http://www.osteopathic.org/inside-aoa/development/aoa-board-certification/Pages/osteopathic-continuous-certification.aspx.
3. AOA Staff. "AOA Statement on Physician-Led Care, Physician Assistant Title Change, and Non-Physician Clinician Use of the Title 'Doctor.'" American Osteopathic Association, May 28, 2021, https://osteopathic.org/2021/05/28/aoa-statement-on-physician-led-care-physician-assistant-title-change-and-non-physician-clinician-use-of-the-title-doctor/.

What Is the American Board of Physician Specialties (ABPS)?

The ABPS® is the official certifying body for the American Association of Physician Specialists (AAPS). However, while it offers board certifications to MDs and DOs, I want to caution against confusing these with the certifications provided by member specialties recognized by the ABMS or the AOA, even if they are acknowledged by the Centers for Medicare and Medicaid Services, the Veterans Administration (VA), and the US Armed Forces, along with specific advertising rules.

The ABPS certifies physicians who may have not obtained qualifications and certifications in specialties and subspecialties recognized by the ABMS or AOA, as well as in specialties unique to this association.

ABPS member boards are recognized only in some states. California prohibits physicians from advertising that they are "board certified" if their certification comes from a board recognized solely by the ABPS unless they are also certified by a member board of the ABMS or AOA. A similar situation may exist in New York or your state; check, as approximately twenty states have established specific rules for AAPS members regarding advertising.

The ABPS provides certifications in:

- Administrative Medicine
- Anesthesiology
- Dermatology
- Diagnostic Radiology
- Disaster Medicine
- Emergency Medicine
- Family Medicine Obstetrics
- Family Medicine
- General Surgery
- Geriatric Medicine
- Hospital Medicine
- Integrative Medicine
- Internal Medicine
- Obstetrics and Gynecology
- Ophthalmology
- Orthopedic Surgery
- Plastic Surgery
- Psychiatry
- Radiation Oncology
- Urgent Care Medicine

Notice that it includes specialties of questionable validity, such as integrative medicine and disaster medicine, where residencies may not qualify a candidate for recognition by any of the ABMS or AOA. Metabolic medicine and anti-aging medicine have been under consideration for membership in this association.

The ABPS recognition of integrative medicine as a board should speak for itself. Remember that "integrative" is the term added to alternative and complementary health care, and it pertains to CAIH, which I already mentioned seems akin to quackery to me.

I inherently distrust any specialist claiming to be certified by a board recognized only by the ABPS. I'm particularly suspicious of the ethics of those who promote themselves using certifications not recognized by the ABMS or the AOA. But that's just my perspective.

References and Recommended Reading

1. "The American Board of Physician Specialties," Wikipedia, https://en.wikipedia.org/wiki/American_Board_of_Physician_Specialties. American Board of Physician Specialties Webpage. Accessed 13 Dec 2022
2. American Board of Physician Specialties, accessed on April 12, 2024, https://www.abpsus.org/abps/.

Who Is a Mid-Level Provider?

The term "mid-level practitioner" encompasses several roles within healthcare. Synonyms for mid-level practitioners include non-physician providers (NPP) and advanced practice providers (APP). I prefer a term I coined: "mid-medically educated provider (MEP)."

I also dislike the term "advanced" practice provider because I find it misleading. Mid-level practitioners may have taken on more responsibilities than non-providers, such as nurses, but they do not have an advanced scope of practice compared to physicians. Therefore, I ask, compared to whom do they consider themselves advanced? Certainly not MDs or DOs.

Using APP to refer to advanced practice providers creates significant confusion for patients. I read a report about a patient who called an office and specifically didn't want to see the physicians. He preferred to see the PA because she was identified as the "advanced practice provider." Naturally, the patient wanted to be seen by the most qualified practitioner; however, as you may already have learned, the APP does not possess the same level of education as the medical doctor supervising such a midlevel provider.

Mid-level practitioners traditionally encompass nurse practitioners, physician assistants, nurse anesthetists, anesthesiologist assistants, and nurse midwives. For simplicity, I and many others including doctors and administrators of medical systems collectively refer to them as non-physician providers or NPPs.

The term "mid-level" was developed to reflect their education and level of decision-making. Mid-level providers may be more educated than MAs, some nurses, emergency medical technicians, surgical assistants, and so on, but they do not have an MD or DO education or competence.

NPPs are constantly pushing to invade the field of medicine. The terminologies they fight for are in constant flux, so remain attentive and cautious.

Unfortunately, NPPs and other providers go to Congress instead of medical school to continually challenge the status quo and gain privileges. They do this to see if, through perseverance, politicians seeking votes would support their ability to call themselves doctors without putting in comparable effort to that of MDs and DOs.

One wonders why certain providers, which include APPs, NPs, PAs, chiropractors, and others, wish to be called doctors and prescribe medications. If this is the case, why don't they attend medical school? Part of the answer is likely that it takes too long, is more demanding, is expensive, is inconvenient, requires higher SAT scores, and more.

However, MDs and DOs can do it; therefore, I believe that no one without an MD or DO degree from an accredited medical school should be permitted to prescribe.

Of course, in situations like COVID-19, HIV, monkeypox (now pox—to be politically correct and not offend monkeys—no kidding), chikungunya, Zika, Ebola, and any other public health emergencies that may arise (like now, measles), I would not be outright antagonistic to allowing APPs, including pharmacy doctors (PharmDs), to prescribe and deliver vaccines and a few specific drugs—provided they receive adequate instruction and direction from the government on how to do so and only for a limited time.

The constant lobbying of Congress by mid-level practitioners for privileges, despite their education not being equivalent to that of MDs or DOs, strikes me as ethically inappropriate. For example, as recently as September 15, 2023, nurse practitioners (NPs) sued the state of California for the right to use the "doctor" label despite truth-in-advertising laws in the state.

It frustrates MDs and DOs when members of Congress approve the prescribing practices of mid-level practitioners and pharmacists or grant them other privileges in exchange for votes or favors.

References and Recommended Reading

1. Amy Lynn Sorrel. "'If That's Not Expanding Scope, I Don't Know What Is': Bill Grants Scope Shortcut to Rural Aprns by Amy Lynn Sorrel." Texmed, Texas Medical Association, May 5, 2025, www.texmed.org/Template.aspx?id=66056.
2. AOA Staff. "AOA Statement on Physician-Led Care, Physician Assistant Title Change, and Non-Physician Clinician Use of the Title 'Doctor,'" American Osteopathic Association, May 28, 2021, https://osteopathic.org/2021/05/28/aoa-statement-on-physician-led-care-physician-assistant-title-change-and-non-physician-clinician-use-of-the-title-doctor/.
3. Sarah Dlc-Tanner. @flossytoothglossy. "SB 24-194 Was Signed Into Law." Instagram, May 6, 2025. https://www.instagram.com/p/DJS2KWHsIcY/?utm_source=ig_web_button_share_sheet
4. Tanya Albert Henry, "Nurse Practitioners Sue for Right to Use 'Doctor' Label," American Medical Association, September 15, 2023, https://www.ama-assn.org/practice-management/scope-practice/nurse-practitioners-sue-right-use-doctor-label.

Who Is a Physician Assistant or "Associate" (PA)?

Physician assistants (PAs) are, or should be, integral members of a physician's team. They were meant to assist MDs and DOs in providing care for patients.

Their trade was initially designed to assist, hence the name, not to replace MDs and DOs in examining patients; in ordering laboratory and imaging tests and more, intended to diagnose and treat patients; in performing tasks like intubations in the ER or the intensive care unit, and in performing catheterizations (of the urinary tract) under the jurisdiction of a supervising physician.

However, that is different from what occurred in the long run. Nowadays, PAs serve as substitutes for physicians, occasionally impersonating them.

By seeking to change their title from physician assistant to physician associate, they demonstrate an attempt to imply that they have obtained a higher level of medical education without substantially increasing their studies.

PAs do not undergo the same medical school programs designed for MDs or DOs. Technically (according to a definition established by the Social Security Administration), they are not considered "real" physicians. While some PA programs are affiliated with medical schools, others are offered at community colleges and hospital-based "institutes, " such as the Massachusetts General Hospital Institute of Health, which specialize in delivering various professional degrees, many of which are covered in this book.

PAs are currently grouped with NPs and other healthcare providers in the category known as non-physician providers (NPP), "mid-level," or "extender"—terms many of them dislike. I refer to them as mid-educated providers or MEPs, which they will undoubtedly dislike even more. The fact is that none of them seem to know what they do not know.

The name of their trade, either by accident, creative marketing, or a lack of legal oversight, implies that PAs are indeed "physicians" who assist with some of the tasks performed by MDs and DOs. PAs are assistants to the physicians they work for at a higher level than medical assistants (MAs) or nurses that are not NPs.

The Accreditation Review Commission on Education for the Physician Assistant (ARC-PA) is the organization that defines and evaluates the education standards for PAs. It exists to protect the interests of PAs and the public. To be licensed as a PA, one must graduate from programs at schools accredited by the ARC-PA.

Currently, PA programs are at the master's level, requiring applicants to hold an undergraduate degree. They were previously two-year associate programs and later four-year undergraduate programs.

A GPA of 3.0 is considered "competitive" for entry (compare that to around 4.0 for MDs) into PA programs. Candidates may transfer other experiences, such as education in health care, including nursing, military medicine, and paramedic practice, among others. The traditional entrance exam has been the GRE, with typical scores for those admitted to PA programs hovering around the 50th percentile. An increasing number of programs are using a new PA College Admissions Test (PA-CAT), which is more similar in content to the MCAT.

Then, they can attend one of the ARC-PA accredited PA programs, which lasts twenty-eight months or just over two years, to be awarded the PA, a master's level degree.

After this, PAs must pass a certifying test given by the Physician Assistant National Certifying Exam (PANCE) administered by the National Commission on Certification of Physician Assistants (NCCPA). This five-hour exam consists of five one-hour blocks with sixty questions in each block. These questions are typically straightforward recall or basic diagnostic, so-called "first order" questions. Passing it allows them to add a -C to their PA (PA-C).

PA candidates can be trained in accredited programs at academic medical centers, but these must not be mistaken as going through medical school, even if located in the same building.

PA programs last two to three years and integrate classroom and clinical studies. Therefore, they are completed in roughly six to seven years, including college, which is about one-third to one-half the time it takes for a doctoral candidate to become an MD or DO.

Due to the time constraints, PA training is not as deep, intense, or academically rigorous as that of MDs or DOs. Just look at their on-call schedules. A local university had a freeway sign promoting PA education online, stating, "without the need to touch a single patient." No internship or residency is required.

PA training can be completed in a similar time frame as an NP degree. Both professionals are regarded as mid-level providers.

In their favor against NPs, PAs argue that doctors provide their training, whereas NPs obtain it from other nurses. Consequently, PAs assert that their training and knowledge are superior. As you might expect, NPs assert the contrary.

PAs apply for state licensure with the NCCPA. PAs can take a recertification board exam every ten years.

Some PAs seem inclined to pose as medical doctors, basking in the confusion their title confers on patients. This becomes evident when one reads the bulletins of state medical societies that oversee medical practice and penalize fraudulent behaviors, sometimes revoking licenses. Call a PA "doctor" and see if they will correct you.

At a practice where I once worked, a PA attempted to present herself as a "board-certified dermatologist." The ABMS and the AOA designate this title exclusively for an MD or DO who has completed an internship and a three-year residency in dermatology and has passed the rigorous certifying exam, never for a mid-level practitioner.

The PA had convinced an appointment clerk to tell patients that she, not unlike her supervising dermatologist, had such board certification. After investigating, we discovered she had taken a weekend course and obtained a "certificate of attendance." After the discovery, she was forbidden to claim such misleading certification. She was eventually fired for a couple of egregious medical errors.

I often hear patients refer to PAs at other practices as "doctors," particularly- though not exclusively- after visiting one of those "docs in the box" settings (sometimes located inside pharmacies) where they seek quick, convenient medical attention or to practices where the supervising MD or DO is not visible.

Medical practices today employ NPPs to treat more patients per hour without the added expense of an MD or DO. In other words, practices bring in mid-level providers to generate more revenue, although they might claim it is "to provide better care and increase access to the community."

Despite their reduced training, insurers and other third-party payers, including government entities, compensate practices similarly or, in some areas, slightly less (about 85%) than what an MD or DO would agree to accept for work performed by an NPP.

In 2018, indirect billing- where services provided by mid-levels are billed under the name of an MD or DO- cost Medicare nearly $200 million.

I use the following scenario in my presentations and discussions with peers who hire mid-levels: "If you are a dermatologist in another state and your granddaughter is referred by a pediatrician to a dermatologist to assess the risk of a pigmented lesion growing on her scalp, and your daughter later tells you that the dermatologist could not see the baby, but that the practice's PA or NP told her not to worry, would you feel at ease or tell your daughter to return the child to be examined by the supervising dermatologist?" Invariably, the answer is: "Send the baby back or go to another dermatologist." To them, I reply, "If the midlevel report is not trustworthy enough for your granddaughter, why should it be good enough for any of your patients?"

However, realistically speaking, the horses are out of the barn, and a lasso to bring them back is missing. Since they have become a fixture in medical offices, urgent care facilities, and similar environments, we should educate NPPs as effectively as possible and help them learn how to collaborate appropriately with supervising MDs and DOs. Our goal is to prevent misdiagnosis, mistreatment, and harm to patients. Remember the words of D. H. Lawrence: "What the eye doesn't see and the mind doesn't know doesn't exist."

A study revealed that PAs perform disproportionately more biopsies of pigmented lesions compared to dermatologists. At the same time, although requiring fewer biopsies, dermatologists diagnose more melanomas, one of the most lethal types of skin lesions that should not be overlooked. As a result, many dermatologists hold the well-supported belief that when NPPs are uncertain about a lesion, they tend to send it to the lab instead of bringing it to their supervising physician's attention, possibly out of embarrassment. Therefore, when in doubt, cut it out. However, since there are risks associated with biopsies, even if minor, this procedure should only be performed when necessary.

My recommendation is to seek care from MDs or DOs rather than, at least initially and periodically, from medically mid-medically educated providers (MEPs) or extenders.

As patients, we all have the right to request, if not demand, to be checked by a full-fledged medical doctor at any or all visits. After all, the service will most likely be billed as if an MD or DO perform it. Physicians may delegate some follow-up and treatments to a PA with the patient's consent, but the plan should always be laid out and followed by the supervising MD or DO after the physician has made the diagnosis.

PAs, envying NPs, are relentlessly pushing in Congress for the right to prescribe unsupervised, and in a few states, they may have gotten such a privilege. Again, caveat emptor!

Recently, one of the big health insurers finally wised up and reduced payments for services by mid-levels by 15 percent. Many of their services are billed under the doctor who supervises them. Then, for some reason, it had to backtrack on the plan.

References and Recommended Reading

1. American Academy of Physician Assistants, www.aapa.org.
2. "Occupational Outlook Handbook: Physician Assistants," Bureau of Labor Statistics, US Department of Labor, http://www.bls.gov/ooh/healthcare/physician-assistants.htm.
3. James F. Crawley, "Physician Assistants and Their Role in Primary Care, *Virtual Mentor*. 2012;5:411–414, https://journalofethics.ama-assn.org/article/physician-assistants-and-their-role-primary-care/2012-05.
4. "2021 Statistical Profile of Certified PAs: Annual Report," National Commission on Certification of Physician Assistants, https://www.nccpa.net/wp-content/uploads/2022/08/2021 StatProfileofCertifiedPAs-A-3.2.pdf.
5. Victoria Bailey, "Eliminating Indirect Billing for NPs and PAs Could Save Medicare $194M," TechTarget, June 14, 2022, https://www.techtarget.com/revcyclemanagement/news/366600826/Eliminating-Indirect-Billing-for-NPs-PAs-Could-Save-Medicare-194M.

Who Is a Nurse Practitioner (NP)?

NPs are nurses with advanced degrees in nursing. Advanced nursing studies encompass nurses who specialize as clinical specialists, midwives, informatics experts, educators, leaders in administration, and practitioners. Additional degrees are introduced periodically.

Advanced (and we previously discussed the usage of the term "advanced") nurses are, or should be, an essential part of the medical team. Like PAs, they should strive to enhance the outcomes that physicians intend to provide. However, some NPs believe they are competent enough to establish practices independently, without MD or DO supervision—on their own—which I find hazardous.

The American Academy of Nurse Practitioners, the NPs advocacy organization, stated that NPs should be able to practice healthcare independently without needing a consulting or supervising physician. Obviously, they don't know what they don't know.

Despite significant differences in education, scope of practice, prescribing authority, and independent setups, NPs belong to the categories of MEPs with other NPP, which includes PAs.

The salaries of NPs and PAs are similar or slightly in favor of PAs for reasons that probably have to do with politics and economics more than education.

The levels of nursing training are:

1. Licensed practical nurse (LPN) or licensed vocational nurse (LVN) (one-year program)
2. Nurse associate (two-year program conferring eligibility to become a registered nurse)
3. Registered nurse (RN) (two- to four-year programs to confer eligibility for a bachelor's degree in nursing (RN/BSN) or a master of science in nursing (RN/MSN)
4. Nurse practitioner (NP) or advanced practice registered nurse (APRN) requires at least an MSN
5. RN with a doctorate in nursing and other fields (PhD, DNP)

A PhD in nursing or DNP should not be confused with a doctorate in medicine, as often happens to their delight.

A California NP was charged with referring to herself as a "doctor" and repeatedly failing to clarify that she was an NP. Despite being found reprimandable, she continued to deny any wrongdoing, asserting that she should be able to call herself "a doctor" to her patients without needing to specify in what field (nursing), a stance supported by some NP organizations.

Nurses can progress from one level to the next by adding a year or two to their previous level of education or directly entering dedicated programs that can take them to the desired level.

For example, by following the first path, an LVN can choose to become an RN, and an RN can choose to become an NP; each advancement requires one to two additional years of study through "bridge programs." Alternatively, using the second path, they can enroll in a nursing program that awards an RN, BSN, and MSN.

NPs are RNs who further their training by obtaining a master's degree with a specific focus on a population. Currently, eight population foci are recognized by various nursing accreditation agencies: family, acute care adult-gerontology, primary care adult-gerontology, emergency, women's health, pediatrics, neonatology, and psychiatric and mental health. These focuses define their scope of practice. The intent of individual NPs to work in medical specialties that do not align with their population focus should be interpreted with caution.

A family NP program that only offers a superficial understanding of preventive primary care services may not adequately prepare an NP to work exclusively (and certainly not independently) in fields such as dermatology, rheumatology, and cardiology, among others.

Nursing students can enroll in accelerated programs that advance them to the master's or doctoral level within one to five years. However, in general, it takes six to seven years to become a nurse practitioner (NP), which is somewhat comparable to the training required for a physician assistant (PA).

A college admission test, such as the SAT or the American College Test (ACT), is often required for acceptance into a pre-nursing or direct-entry nursing program at a college or university. Those who are accepted into a pre-nursing program typically take the Test of Essential Academic Skills (TEAS) before being fully admitted to a nursing program.

To become licensed and work as RNs, they must complete nursing coursework, clinical rotations, and achieve a passing score on the National Council Licensure Examination (NCLEX).

Candidates for NP typically need a bachelor's degree. For those who are not RNs, there are combined "direct-entry" RN-NP programs, where students spend a year earning an accelerated BSN to obtain their RN. After completing this, they dedicate one to two years to earn their MSN and become an NP.

Patients should familiarize themselves with the curricula of potential providers' programs. Many NP programs offer only a single-semester pathophysiology class and another single-semester pharmacology class. The rest of the degree completion time is spent on management, lobbying, and "nursing theory."

NP students usually need to complete 500 to 700 clinical hours, which amounts to about three months of full-time work at forty hours per week. Unlike MDs or DOs, NP students might be tasked with finding their own rotations. They may also have to compensate preceptors who might not be keen on teaching in order to have those hours approved.

NP students may gain hands-on experience, just as medical or PA students do. However, they may end up shadowing physicians for 500 clinical learning hours, which might not align with the "population focus" of their degree. One can easily find "family NP" students accumulating their clinical hours at urology or dermatology offices instead of at a more relevant family medicine clinic.

Don't overlook that the requirements to enter NP schools are less stringent than those for MD or DO programs. The duration of nursing training, even to reach the NP level, is much shorter (and less in-depth), totaling about six versus twelve years. Keep in mind that some master's and doctorate programs in nursing and physician assistant studies are offered online and may not require patient contact!

DNP students can choose to attend doctoral programs, but these do not change their population focus, enhance their clinical skills, or alter their scope of practice. These degrees can be completed entirely online and do not include bedside clinical education, seemingly serving only to earn a title. A notably vocal NP advocate revealed that 85 percent of DNP programs were "non-clinical."

To practice as an NP, individuals must pass a nationally recognized certification exam. NP certifications are challenging because there can be too many "cooks in the kitchen." Family NPs and primary care adult-gerontology NPs may take their certifying exams from the American Academy of Nurse Practitioners (AANP) or the American Nurses Credentialing Center (ANCC). A prospective NP might fail the AANP exam and then pass the ANCC exam the following week (or vice versa)! This scenario is not just hypothetical; it has happened, raising the question: if a particular student can fail one test and pass another, which test should be considered the appropriate standard for clinical practice?

The content of NP licensing exams differs significantly from that of medical licensing exams. While the exams for MDs or DOs typically include questions about diagnosis, treatment, and interpretation of scientific literature, NP licensing exams may encompass nursing-level theory. The clinical practice questions aim to enhance variations in clinical care, dictate practice decisions, protect nurses from legal liability, and serve as a guide for best practices. Reviews to ensure core competency, force field analysis, and risk analysis are conducted by colleagues of the same level of training. However, the questions lack complexity and seem inadequate for assessing the knowledge necessary for independent practice.

Once they graduate, and typically once licensed, NPs may enroll in "fellowships" or "residencies," which have names that seem interchangeable with those used by MDs and DOs. However, many of the programs offered by independent hospitals are not recognized even by nurse credentialing services because they lack a structured curriculum or guidelines. Some "residencies" may not include book learning or written examinations. They are nothing like the ACGME-sanctioned tests for physician residencies and may require no more than thirty-six to forty hours per week (compared to sixty to eighty-plus hours per week in physician residency programs).

NPs may take examinations administered by nursing guilds, such as the Dermatology Nurse Practitioner Certification Board (DNPCB). To qualify as "certified dermatology nurse practitioner," NPs must report 3000 hours or three years of dermatology experience to this private organization. It is unclear what verification process the DNCPB uses to confirm those hours. Applicants must also take a 175-question exam, of which at least 74 percent must be answered correctly to pass. The questions are not authored by dermatologists, and the NPs are not tested at the level of these specialists. Instead, NPs are tested at the level of a dermatology nurse. This type of certification is not recognized by state nursing boards either for initial licensure or recertification since there is no structured curriculum, and it relies on self-reported hours. The nursing field seems inundated with phony guilds and boards.

The oversight of nursing specialties is complex (intentionally, I believe), and some aspects are beyond the scope of this book. The Dermatology Nurse Practitioner Certification Board is "accredited" by the Accreditation Board for Specialty Nursing Certification, an agency for the National Council of State Boards of Nursing's APRN Certification Review Program.

The National Council of State Boards of Nursing administers the NCLEX licensing examination for RNs, but it does not oversee any of the APRN licensing exams for recognized population foci.

Only three of five organizations that administer licensing exams for APRNs are "accredited" by the Accreditation Board for Specialty Nursing Certification, while two others are not. The Accreditation Board states that it has standards for certification, but these standards are not clearly communicated. An application for accreditation appears to be little more than a letter of intent.

To make matters more confusing, there is an American Board of Nursing Specialties, which, in fine print, clarifies that it does not administer certification programs. Although these organizations mention "nursing specialties," they only reference some physician specialties, such as oncology and dermatology, not nursing specialties, like wound care, intubations, catheterizations, and venous line placements. This Board may resemble the ABPS I wrote about in a previous chapter.

Are you completely confused? You should be, because I am as well. The intent of the NPs seems to be ensnaring the public and legislators in a web that delays and leaves investigations into credentialing unexamined. Layers of complexity also serve to extract money from nurses, who must pay one organization after another to feel eligible for licensing.

More than half of states permit NPs to prescribe medications without direct supervision from an MD or DO. I strongly oppose this, yet congressmen seem to think otherwise. They believe they know better. Rest assured, congressmen and their family members likely seek care from MDs or DOs, not NPs or other midlevel practitioners.

Many NPs view themselves as capable of operating independently and establishing offices by themselves, thus pushing the boundaries of their trade into MD or DO territory. They do this at the expense of participating in teams with real medical doctors, whom NPs now pretend to call "collaborators" (like PAs wishing to be called "associates" those MDs or DOs who they work for) instead of supervising physicians. What one group accomplishes in Congress, the other goes for, too.

The public may believe that a given NP is an MD or DO if they introduce themselves as "doctor such-and-such." This can occur if they obtain a DNP or PhD in nursing, anesthesia, or public health and fail to clarify, as it is mandated, that their doctorate, if they hold one, is not in medicine. I have witnessed NPs (and PAs) steer conversations to avoid explaining that their doctorate is not equivalent to those held by MDs or DOs.

Remember that in earlier chapters, I explained that the usurped prefix "Dr." may be displayed on small plaques pinned above the pocket of a uniform, the lapel of a jacket, or even embroidered on a lab coat, followed by the person's name. If the name is not followed by MD or DO, the public and patients should not assume they are being cared for by a medical doctor. This is often seen in television and other visual media advertisements.

Although it may be legal in certain states for NPs to work independently, order tests, and even write prescriptions, my stance is more nuanced: according to the American Academy of Family Physicians, NPs should "function in harmony in an integrated practice arrangement under the direction and responsible supervision of a practicing, licensed physician."

I'll share a funny little story: I sat next to a lady identified as an NP working for a large organization of independently practicing nurses at a recent medical meeting. When I asked who supervises her activities (to see if I had met them), she replied, irked, "We do not need to be supervised as if we were PAs; we use collaborating physicians." Well, not so funny; she clearly didn't realize what she didn't know. "Collaborator" is another linguistic twist intended for self-aggrandizement, self-promotion, and self-adulation purposes.

These cats, too, are out of the bag, and I don't see any nets to bring them back for now.

Some institutions rely on NPs to provide patient care. As a faculty member at a university hospital, I am affiliated with the intensive care unit (ICU), which has MDs and DOs effectively working together with NPs as a highly functional team. During my rotation in the cardiac care unit (CCU), I learned a great deal from the nurses and recognize their value.

In the US, we need about 10,000 MDs; therefore, without NPs, many practices and hospitals would not have enough nighttime coverage. There is no doubt that NPs can perform valuable work. I'm pleased to see them in supervised settings like our ICU, but I have reservations about them working independently or prescribing on their own. A recent report dispelled the notion that the need for more medical doctors is being adequately replaced with NPs and PAs.

Hiring NPPs for urgent care and emergency rooms makes sense to bean counters (not to me). This may explain why we see NPs and PAs in clinics, pharmacies, supermarkets, airports, and even medical offices. I wager the owners' goal is not to provide enhanced quality medical services," as they may claim, but to do so cheaply and profitably.

Believe it or not, the so-called Affordable Care Act (Obamacare) includes a provision that protects NPs and PAs from malpractice lawsuits if they work at certain large pharmacy chains, such as CVS and Walgreens. This is based on the premise that genuine doctor-patient relationships are not established, even when these extenders operate in the same capacity as a licensed physician with an MD or DO degree. Be aware that you would be on your own in those settings. Don't complain later, as I told you so.

If you are receiving care from an NP, you can and should request to meet the supervising or "collaborating" MD or DO. Otherwise you are not being wise, and someone else may be having your cake and eating it too.

Be informed that a profession that imitates NP's invasion of the medical turf is being created—this one is invading the dentists: dental therapists (DTs). I've been reading about this for about a few years, but it appears that it wasn't until just now that dentists became concerned and started fighting them back. Keep your dentist a DDS or DDM. There is even a push to have "veterinary professional associates (VPAs)" diagnosing and performing surgery on pets rather than a qualified veterinarian (who holds a doctorate in veterinary medicine, or DVM)!

References and Recommended Reading

1. "Nurse Practitioners," American Academy of Family Physicians, http://www.aafp.org/about/policies/all/nurse-practitioners.html.
2. Doctors, Inc., "When the Nurse Wants to Be Called 'Doctor,'" *The New York Times*, October 1, 2011, https://www.nytimes.com/2011/10/02/health/policy/02docs.html.
3. "A Guide to the Different Types of Nursing Degrees, " All Nursing Schools, http://www.allnursingschools.com/nursing-careers/article/nursing-program-types/.
4. Diana Furchtgott-Roth, "CVS and Walgreens Get a Helping Hand from Obama," MarketWatch, https://www.marketwatch.

com/story/cvs-walgreens-get-helping-hand-from-obama-2014-04-11.
5. Nurse.org.Staff. "Types of Master's in Nursing (MSN) Degree | Programs 2025," Nurse.org, https://nurse.org/education/ultimate-list-masters-degrees-nursing/.
6. "Nurse Practitioner vs. Physician Assistant," Wikipedia, accessed in December 2023.

Who Is a Nurse Anesthetist (CRNA)? An Anesthesiologist Assistant? An Anesthesiologist?

Anesthetists are providers of anesthesia. They help during surgery and other procedures, like electroconvulsive therapy, brain injury, or coma, all of which may be painful and stressful.

The term anesthesia refers to a lack of sensation, especially in relation to pain (in Greek, 'a' means without, and 'esthesia' means sensation).

The traditionally recognized medical anesthesia provider is the anesthesiologist with an MD or DO degree, who should not be confused with the nurse anesthetist.

Currently, some specialized nurses with master's-level certification can provide anesthesia, although their scope is limited. These nurses are known as certified registered nurse anesthetists (CRNAs). There is a strong push to convert their programs to doctorate-level, culminating in a Doctorate in Nurse Anesthesia

Practice (DNAP). (This seems to be another degree attempting to claim the title of "doctor" in clinical practice.)

CRNA candidates start as licensed RNs or BSNs and are typically required to have a year of experience in an acute care setting, such as an intensive care unit (ICU), before entering a two-year accredited advanced nursing program that prepares them for the certifying exam. The doctoral programs include a year of clinical rotations assisting in anesthesia and practicing under the supervision of a licensed CRNA or anesthesiologist.

There has been a movement among CRNA organizations and students in nurse anesthesia programs to refer to the final year of clinical rotations as a "residency." It is important to note that residency in every other medical or allied health field refers to postgraduate practical training under a licensed supervisor in a discipline. Residency for physicians, pharmacists, psychologists, and others is not the same as clinical rotations undertaken by students who are still enrolled and paying tuition. Therefore, do not be misled by so-called nurse anesthesia residents. They are students who cannot and should not work independently or unsupervised.

The entire training process for a CRNA may take six to seven years, starting from nursing school. In contrast, the training of anesthesiologists, who are MDs or DOs, lasts twelve years: four years of pre-medical education, four years in medical school, followed by an internship year, and then three years in residency to qualify for board certification in anesthesiology. This duration does not include an optional year or two for fellowship. In summary, CRNAs require half the years compared to anesthesiologists.

Anesthesiologist assistants (AAs) are another category of mid-level providers in the field of anesthesia. They hold a role similar to that of CRNAs. While CRNAs typically earn an undergraduate degree in nursing, AAs generally complete pre-medical or science degrees. AAs undergo twenty-eight months of anesthesia training. The first year focuses on foundational knowledge, including anatomy, physiology, radiology, and pharmacology as it relates to anesthesia. During the second year, AAs participate in hands-on clinical rotations, assisting with anesthesia in various departments. Graduates of these programs receive a Master of Medical Science degree in anesthesiology. There are only a few AA programs available across the country, and only a limited number of states license AAs, primarily due to insufficient lobbying efforts and competition from the CRNA lobby.

In addition to putting people to sleep for surgery and other procedures, anesthesiologists with MD or DO degrees may operate pain clinics and ICUs, where they can prescribe medications as needed. This responsibility stems from their extensive education and training through medical school, residency, and optional fellowships.

In most countries, anesthesiologists are the only professionals authorized to administer anesthesia. In the US, some states allow CRNAs to provide anesthesia without the direct supervision of an anesthesiologist, although the relative safety of patients solely in the care of CRNAs is, questionably, and I think, not as secure.

Publications funded by the American Association of Nurse Anesthetists may lead one to believe that the death risk associated with anesthesia administered by unsupervised CRNAs is similar to that provided by anesthesiologists, even acknowledging that they handle less complex cases.

Publications in response sponsored by the American Society of Anesthesiologists identified biases in those studies and reported increases in complications and mortality when anesthetists worked without supervision from anesthesiologists.

A study funded by the Agency for Healthcare Research and Quality found that the presence of anesthesiologists prevented more than six deaths per 1000 cases of complications arising from surgery or anesthesia.

The American Society of Anesthesiologists believes that legislation and regulations enabling CRNAs to work independently stem from acquiring their degrees through political means. So, what's new?

Once again, similar to other NPPs, Elvis has left the building. Many hospitals, surgical centers, and other facilities depend on CRNAs to administer anesthesia, especially in rural areas where the arrival of an anesthesiologist may be delayed.

My son was scheduled for knee surgery. The evening before the procedure, a very pleasant CRNA introduced herself as the one who would administer his anesthesia and needed to ask a few questions. I informed her, as delicately as possible, that I preferred a board-certified anesthesiologist to handle it. She understood and left. Problem solved. You can do the same. For a cataract surgery on me, I was comfortable with a CRNA administering mine. That illustrates how I feel about CRNAs versus anesthesiologists well enough. However, that occurred under ideal circumstances.

References and Recommended Reading

1. "Become a CNRA," American Association of Nurse Anesthetists, https://www.aana.com/about-us/about-crnas/become-a-crna/.

2. Epstein J, "Nurse Anesthetists Don't Measure Up," *The Ledger*, July 2, 2013, https://www.theledger.com/story/news/2013/07/02/nurse-anesthetists-dont-measure-up/26851351007/.
3. Karen S. Sibert, "Unsupervised Anesthesia Care by a Nurse Anesthetist Is a Threat to Patient Safety," KevinMD.com, November 17, 2011, https://kevinmd.com/2011/11/unsupervised-anesthesia-care-nurse-anesthetist-threat-patient-safety.html.

Who Is a Midwife? An Obstetrician (OB/GYN)?

Midwives are healthcare providers who help women during labor and delivery and the pre- and post-partum periods. Their care may start during the family planning stages. Many midwives work at birthing centers or at clients' homes, while others work in hospitals or are affiliated with them.

Midwives primarily care for healthy pregnant women whose deliveries are expected to be uncomplicated. Although some midwives' have extensive and specialized training, they are not medical doctors specializing in obstetrics and gynecology (OB/GYN).

There are three kinds of midwives:

1. Certified midwife
2. Certified professional midwife
3. Certified nurse midwife (CNM)

The first two are permitted to practice in only some states, while CNMs can practice in all states, including Washington, DC.

Typically, all midwives undergo midwifery training and complete the certifying examination.

To become a CNM, the process is one of advanced nursing practice (ANP), like the one described for NPs, who evolve from RN/BSN to their midwife degree through a master's-level instructional program.

This process can take five to eight years from the start of nursing school. For reference, it takes at least twelve years to become an OB/GYN, as they are required to first be an MD or DO, which takes four years. This is followed by a one-year internship and then three years of supervised obstetrics and gynecology to qualify for board certification. This is an arduous, lengthy, and intense process where many hours are spent in the training hospital.

Midwifery websites refer higher-risk patients to OB/GYN physicians, including women with diabetes, high blood pressure, kidney disease, epilepsy, heart disease, active infections, and other conditions that may increase risks during pregnancy, labor and delivery, and the neonatal period.

For my family, I would seek care from an OB/GYN at a well-equipped hospital where a perinatologist, a doctor specializing in managing complications that can occur around delivery, could be found.

After completing the aforementioned training to become an OB/GYN, a perinatologist is an MD or DO who undergoes an additional two-to-three-year fellowship in maternal-fetal medicine. This amounts to more than fifteen years of education and training!

Perinatologists care for women who are undergoing in vitro fertilization, are pregnant with multiples, have placental abnormalities, show atypical screening results, experience injuries during pregnancy, have suffered multiple miscarriages, require chemotherapy or immunotherapy, or use controlled substances during pregnancy. They also attend to those with a history of prematurity, carry one or more underweight embryos, suffer from preeclampsia, have predicted genetic abnormalities, and face various other factors that increase the risks associated with pregnancy and delivery.

During my medical school years and internship, I cared for and participated in hundreds of deliveries; thus, I can confidently state that things can "go sour" surprisingly and quickly. A mother experiencing postpartum hemorrhage or a newborn requiring resuscitation is something that should not occur at home or a birthing center, particularly if not connected to a capable hospital.

For my children and grandchildren, even if their mom and dad have no known risks, my choice would undoubtedly be an OB/GYN at a hospital well-equipped to handle deliveries and neonatal complications immediately, knowing that a perinatologist would be within reach at delivery time. I insist!

References and Recommended Reading

1. "What Is a Midwife?" Midwives Alliance, http://mana.org/about-midwives/what-is-a midwife.
2. "Comparison of Certified Nurse-Midwives, Certified Midwives, and Certified Professional Midwives," Midwife, http://www.midwife.org/ACNM/files/ccLibraryFiles/Filename/000000001385CNM%20CM%20CPM%ComparisonChart%20082511.pdf.
3. Jeffrey Kluger, "Doctors versus Midwives: The Birth Wars Rage On," *Time*, May 16, 2009, https://time.com/archive/6933514/doctors-versus-midwives-the-birth-wars-rage-on/.
4. "What Is a Perinatologist, and What Do They Do?" Healthline.com, http://healthline.comhealth/baby/what-is-a-perinatologist#why-to-see-one.

Who Is a "Foot Doctor," a Podiatrist, a Doctor of Podiatric Medicine (DPM)?

A podiatrist with a doctorate in podiatric medicine, or DPM, specializes in foot and ankle healthcare.

DPMs diagnose and treat callouses, corns, plantar warts, ingrown toenails, feet and toenail fungus, bunions, heel spurs, arch problems, foot infections, and injuries.

Before entering podiatry school, candidates must complete college courses that include biology, inorganic and organic chemistry, physics, anatomy, physiology, genetics, psychology, sociology, and English. They must maintain a C average and achieve a GPA between 2.5 and 3, depending on the school (note that the GPA required for MD school is typically closer to 4).

Then, they may take the MCAT®, hoping for a high enough score to gain admission into podiatry school. My search for the appropriate score was complicated, mysterious, and troublesome, as many podiatry schools do not specify their acceptable minimum on their websites. An average score of

494 kept appearing. It must be above 500 to be accepted into most MD schools; in fact, it must be above 512 to get into the better ones (I have some doubts about that 494 being accurate; it seems too high to me).

Podiatry students spend four years in school, with the first two years dedicated to basic sciences such as microbiology, anatomy, pathology, chemistry, and pharmacology. After completing these two years of didactic courses, students must take their version of the board exam known as the American Podiatric Medical Licensing Examination (APMLE) Part 1. The following two years focus on rotating through private practices, didactic clinics, and hospitals to develop clinical skills in podiatry. During the fourth year, they are required to take APMLE® Part 2. Graduates of podiatry school earn a degree in podiatry.

Afterward, most pursue a three-year residency program, typically hospital-based, where they train in surgery and clinical practice. While the structure of their training may resemble that of an MD or DO, it is not identical nor conducted with the same rigor.

The US's Council on Podiatric Medical Education accredits less than twenty podiatry colleges.

I am fond of podiatrists because they undergo a lengthy and demanding higher education process. However, theirs is not the medical school from which MDs and DOs graduate.

Yet, they found a way to refer to themselves as "foot doctors," "foot and ankle doctors," and similar titles without undergoing the rigorous training typical of MDs and DOs. Some may assert that they attended "medical school" while conveniently neglecting to mention that they applied to, were accepted at, and graduated from *podiatric* medical school or podiatry school. Although some podiatry programs are affiliated with osteopathic medical schools, they represent a minority.

Some have an issue with podiatrists using the term "(foot) doctor" because they do not graduate from medical schools like those for MDs and DOs. Many are surprised when they are told their "foot doctor" did not attend medical school. The title "foot doctor" has been a source of confusion in the public mind from the moment the permission to use it was granted to podiatrists.

Some podiatrists describe themselves as "diplomats" of the American Boards of Podiatric Surgery, Diabetic Foot Wounds, Limb Salvage, and Podiatric Orthopedics. Unsatisfied podiatrists even go so far as to use the title podiatric medicine doctor (PMD), which, to me, covertly muddies the waters by furthering confusion by having MD as the last two letters in the suffix that follows their name. Clever.

DPMs primarily compete for the turf of orthopedic surgeons, who are indeed MDs or DOs, particularly regarding foot bones, tendons, nerves, and vessels. They also compete for the domain of dermatologists, who must be MDs or DOs working on the skin of the soles, the tops of the feet, toes, and toenails.

I called my favorite orthopedic surgeon, who specializes in feet and ankles, to ask him why searching for "foot and ankle surgeon" yields no board-certified MDs or DOs, only DPMs. He explained that all orthopedic surgeons receive extensive training in foot and ankle surgery during their residency and fellowship, making a specific board certification in the subspecialty unnecessary.

The same applies to dermatology; nobody can beat me at removing a plantar wart, leaving no scar. I, being the dermatologist who literally "wrote the book" on cryotherapy and cryosurgery (the use of liquid nitrogen or other "cold" applications for medical treatment) of the skin. Okay, I bragged.

Despite their busy schedules, many dermatologists would gladly refer patients to DPMs or collaborate with them in the care of foot patients, sharing responsibilities in areas where DPMs excel due to their education, training, equipment, and frequency of encounters. These areas include caring for diabetic feet, trimming excessively thickened and hyper-curved nail plates, managing callouses, and addressing other conditions commonly affecting the elderly.

Many podiatrists work as part of a team at orthopedic practices.

Podiatrists can prescribe orthotics, orthopedic shoes, and braces. They can recommend over-the-counter topical agents, but they cannot prescribe most oral or injectable (systemic) medications. However, they can prescribe a few FDA-approved topical antifungals, treatments for callouses and warts, and creams for ulcer healing, with a few exceptions, but only if it falls within their scope of practice and not in all states. Their limitations in prescribing may change over time.

For example, a podiatrist may be able to prescribe a systemic oral medication like terbinafine to treat tinea pedis or "athlete's foot" because that lies within their turf; however, infections beyond the feet and ankle do not, as they don't have the medical education to treat outside the regions of the foot and ankle. What if there is a drug-induced liver or heart injury from the prescription of an oral antifungal? Podiatrists would have to consult with an MD or DO. Ideally, a hepatologist or a cardiologist, respectively, will be needed to manage the complication. DPMs may be restricted from performing some surgical procedures.

DPMs are required to obtain state licenses to practice in their respective states.

DPMs can obtain certifications from several podiatry boards. The American Board of Podiatric Medicine (ABPM®) is recognized by the American Podiatric Medical Association (APMA) to provide certification in Podiatric Orthopedics and Primary Podiatric Medicine (PO&PPM), which is not recognized by either the ABMS or the AOA.

Some orthopedic surgeons, who may have spent around fourteen years in training, resent DPMs' attempts to encroach upon the domains of foot, ankle, knee, and even hand surgery. Others, however, appear indifferent, trusting that their superior competence, knowledge, and outcomes will speak for themselves.

Orthopedic surgeons reacted to Massachusetts Senate Bill 1216, which attempted to change the language of the law from "foot" to "foot and the ankle." This would have granted DPMs the right to amputate feet, practice surgery on the ankles, and use general anesthesia to perform those and other complicated procedures.

The Massachusetts Medical Society countered that attempt, stating that podiatrists "were not medical school graduates and thus have a different education." Not enough, I interpret.

Paraphrasing one of their arguments, "Amazing successes (in the hands of orthopedic surgeons)…should not imply that ankle surgery is a simple matter…and the qualifications of DPMs do not come close to those of orthopedic surgeons."

In 2010, the Texas Medical Association won an eight-year legal battle against podiatrists that would have permitted DPMs to treat ankle injuries.

Ridiculous attempts by DPMs to invade the area of knee surgery, including joint replacement and, believe it or not, hand surgery, are looming. If orthopedic surgeons and other MDs lower their guard, DPMs may gradually expand their scope of practice to include the skull; consequently, chiropractors performing cranial manipulations will be the ones who are upset.

The children's song "Dem Bones" comes to mind: "The toe bone is connected to the foot bone / the foot bone is connected to the ankle bone / the ankle bone is connected to the leg bone / the leg bone is connected to the knee bone." Funny, if not for concerning.

Some podiatrists sell products in their offices, such as "podiatric Crocs™," "DPM creams," "special soles," and more, to generate extra revenue. However, the effectiveness of their reportedly overpriced soles and inserts may not make them competitive compared to others sold at pharmacies and stores that claim to improve feet and misalignment-related health issues.

Please do not conclude that I don't like DPMs because I do. I respect their trade and am betting that one day, I will personally need their expertise. I appreciate what DPMs work on and how they do it—under most circumstances.

However, just yesterday (as of this writing), a DO student rotating through my residency program described how a DPM she recently worked with removed a small wart in an operating room (OR) using general anesthesia. I would likely have solved the problem in my office using cryosurgery (freezing) at a fraction of the cost and, I bet, with higher success.

Dermatologists like me, who appreciate the contributions of DPMs to our patient's care, gladly refer to those willing to practice within the podiatric scope, as it aligns with the standards of MDs and DOs. The same (referrals to DPMs) applies to internists, vascular surgeons, and all physicians.

Podiatrists should consider partnering in care instead of stepping onto the turf of orthopedic surgery or the toes of any other medical or surgical specialist (puns intended).

References and Recommended Reading

1. American Board of Podiatric Medicine, https://podiatryboard.org.
2. American College of Foot and Ankle Surgeons, www.acfas.org
3. "Position Statement on Total Ankle Replacement Surgery (2009)," American Orthopedic Foot & Ankle Society, http://www.saintalponsus.org/documents/AOFAS-PositionStatement.pdf.
4. "Podiatric Medical Colleges," Council on Podiatric Medical Education, https://www.cpme.org/podiatric-medical-colleges/.
5. Minnesota Board of Podiatric Medicine, https://mn.gov/boards/podiatric-medicine/.
6. "Podiatry School Fact Sheet," Grand Valley State University, August 2022, https://www.gvsu.edu/cms4/asset/8E60AE8A-DD89-F38B-68F611A92AA5D47A/podiatry_school_fact_sheet(2).pdf.

Who Is an "Eye Doctor," an Optometrist (OD), an Optician, or an Ophthalmologist?

When it comes time to examine your eyes, there are three types of providers: opticians, optometrists, and ophthalmologists. Each one plays an essential role in delivering a different level of care and possesses unique education, training, and expertise.

At the first level is the optician, who fits individuals with glasses based on prescriptions written by optometrists and ophthalmologists. They verify lenses, assist with frame choices, and work with contact lenses and other devices to correct vision.

After obtaining a high school diploma, the training for an optician degree takes eight to twelve months; this can be completed online and at theirr own pace.

Applicants who feel prepared may take either the National Opticianry Competency Examination or the American Board of Opticianry. However, the licensing requirements to practice as an optician vary from state to state.

The second level refers to the optometrist or optometry doctor (OD), a healthcare provider trained to test eyesight, identify ocular abnormalities, prescribe corrective lenses, and help patients see more clearly. Optometrists assert that they are, in practical terms, "primary" vision care providers.

Terminologies like "eye doctor" or "optometric physician" often mislead patients into thinking that ODs attend medical school—they do not.

Doctors who attend medical or osteopathy school and specialize in eye care are called ophthalmologists. The MD or DO suffixes clearly identify them; do not confuse DO with OD. Stay alert!

A path to becoming an OD typically involves three years of college. While it is not always required to enter optometry school, most candidates first earn a bachelor's degree.

Optometry schools generally require a minimum overall collegiate GPA of 3.0 (note that this is close to 4 for medical school admission, a very significant difference). The average GPA for students entering higher-ranked programs is 3.5. Recommended prerequisites for optometry school include biology or zoology, mathematics, chemistry, physics, and English. Specific school requirements may include algebra, calculus, anatomy, physiology, organic chemistry, microbiology, statistics, and psychology.

The Optometry Admission Test is required to apply to a four-year program at an optometry school (not a medical school). These schools offer both classroom and clinical training and are accredited by the Council on Optometric Education. There are less than thirty optometry schools in the US.

Afterward, optometry graduates can elect to pursue an optional "residency" year, something resembling a preceptorship with a mentor, typically in a specialty of optometry.

A master's or PhD from a member school (again, not a medical one) recognized by the Association of Schools and Colleges of Optometry in fields such as vision science, public health, or clinical vision research is considered an additional option.

Despite extensive training, the ophthalmologist- not the optometrist- is the most educated professional qualified to diagnose and treat eye diseases. Again, be aware of the big differences between "eye doctors" and ophthalmologists.

I would like to caution patients and readers about the novel use of the title "therapeutic optometrist" and similar terminologies that may mislead the public into believing they are consulting someone who attended and graduated from medical school.

Ophthalmologists represent the third and highest level of eye care providers. As MDs or DOs, they can address a range of issues from minor sight problems easily corrected with glasses, contact lenses, or lasers, including conditions like "red eye," to the most serious concerns such as orbital area infections (cellulitis) and significant conditions like glaucoma, retinal detachment, macular degeneration, and other causes of blindness and death.

Ophthalmologists should appropriately be the specialists consulted for diagnosing and treating eye complications that arise from systemic diseases, including thyroid eye disease, diabetes, high blood pressure, serious infectious diseases like herpes, autoimmune disorders such as lupus, blistering and scarring conditions, macular degeneration, and sarcoidosis, among many others.

Ophthalmologists should be the only professionals permitted to perform complex and delicate surgeries around the orbit, eyelids, and eyeball—including the cornea, retina, irises, and other parts of the eye. This includes corneal transplants, laser reshaping, treatments for retinal cancer, and procedures to correct strabismus (crossed eyes) or amblyopia (lazy eye) in infants, children, and adults.

Ophthalmologists initially complete all requirements to become an MD or DO, followed by an internship and residency, which may subsequently include a fellowship, a subspecialization, or research time (such as in cornea or retina). The three-year residency training in ophthalmology (after a separate one-year internship) equips ophthalmologists to be the leading experts in the medical, procedural, and surgical treatment of the eye and its disorders. This entire process can take twelve to fifteen years. Therefore, it is unsurprising that ophthalmologists are so protective of their field, especially against ODs who often attempt to encroach upon it.

This zeal extends beyond their financial interests; it also aims to protect patients. They worry that patients may end up in the hands of less competent providers.

As technology makes certain corrective surgeries more reliable, it's possible that a technician, perhaps an OD, could one day perform some procedures, hopefully under the guidance and close supervision of an ophthalmologist. I could be comfortable with that eventually.

In some states, optometrists have sought to broaden the scope of their practice to include both laser and non-laser surgery. While laser eye surgery can primarily be a technical procedure, I would not currently allow a non-ophthalmologist to perform it on me.

The need to remain vigilant is exemplified by ongoing legal battles led by ODs over the turf of ophthalmology, utilizing the "Act Relative to the Modernization of Optometric Patient Care." Similar to the situation in podiatry, the Massachusetts Medical Society has opposed this by arguing that optometric education falls short of requirements: "Doctors of Optometry are not Medical Doctors." However, groups like the American Optometric Association persist in lobbying to push legislation such as the "Optometric Equity in Medicaid Act." This infringement (arguably) conceals the intent to blur public perceptions of the differences between ophthalmology practiced by MDs and DOs and optometry practiced by ODs. To illustrate the scale of the problem, between 1997 and 2010, optometrists made forty-six attempts to be granted surgical privileges; fortunately, all were successfully blocked.

Although ophthalmologists win most legal actions initiated by ODs, the latter's perseverance could eventually pay off by distracting or eroding enough of the former's resistance, thereby allowing ODs to lobby circumventing public safety. Since there are 10,000 more optometrists (read: votes) than ophthalmologists, they are likely to tip the balance in their favor during election time in Congress. Be aware of that problem.

A curiosity I have on behalf of patients is: How can ophthalmologists, ODs, and optometrists compete with retailers selling "readers" for under ten dollars when theirs cost forty-five dollars or more at their locations?

I have a three-year-old grandson who, due to excessive time spent in front of electronic tablets, is very farsighted, according to his pediatric ophthalmologist. His prescription often requires adjustments to lenses and frames. I appreciate the quality of the work we trust for the kid's optometric care, even though it took his father three visits to find a competent, caring optician at a store that offered a $100 discount compared to the first two places they visited.

I always advise consulting with an ophthalmologist first when seeking eye care. Remember to look for the suffix MD or DO.

While follow-up visits with optometrists and opticians may be reasonable sometimes, I prefer that they occur under the recommendation, supervision, and periodic consultation of an ophthalmologist.

For now, please don't permit any surgery on the eye and its surroundings (e.g., orbits, lids) or medical treatments for eye diseases to be prescribed or performed by anyone other than an ophthalmologist. We are considering your eyesight for the rest of your life.

I can confidently tell you firsthand, as I just had cataract surgeries and retinal lasering, that it is not something I would trust anyone but an ophthalmologist—preferably one who is subspecialized and experienced.

References and Recommended Reading

1. "Difference between an Ophthalmologist, Optometrist, and Optician," American Association for Pediatric Ophthalmology and Strabismus, https://www.aapos.org/glossary/difference-between-an-ophthalmologist-optometrist-and-optician.
2. EUGEN. (12/14/22) College Search Counseling. "Optometry School Requirements: The Ultimate Guide," https://www.cscscholarship.org/optometry-school-requirements-the-ultimate-guide.
3. General and School-Specific Prerequisites 2020," Association of Schools and Colleges of Optometry https://optometriceducation.org/wp-content/uploads/2020/05/ASCO-Prerequisites-2020-5-1-20.pdf.
4. Shawna Seed, "Eye Doctors: Optometrists and Ophthalmologists," WebMD, http://www.webmd.com/eye-health/eye-doctors-optometrists-ophthalmologists.
5. Kristen E. Schleiter, "Ophthalmologists, Optometrists, and Scope of Practice Concerns," *Virtual Mentor*, 2010;12:941–945, https://journalofethics.ama-assn.org/article/ophthalmologists-optometrists-and-scope-practice-concerns/2010-12.
6. Matt Hasson, "Bill Seeking to Expand Optometrists' 'Scope of Practice' Sparks Debate," *Ocular Surgery News*, Healio.com,

https://www.healio.com/news/ophthalmology/20120331/bill-seeking-to-expand-optometrists-scope-of-practice-sparks-debate.
7. "Optometrists Provoke Ophthalmologists' Ire Over New Surgery Privileges," http://wwww.escrs.org/Publications/Eurotimes/04October/pdf/regmatters.pdf
8. "Grassroots Action Key to Fate Pending AOA-Backed Bills," http://www.aoa.org/Documents/ArchivesMuseum?AOA_News/AOA_News_Volume_45_Number_17_May_28_2007.pdf.
9. "Ophthalmologists Object as Mississippi Panel Approves Bill Expanding Optometry," http://www.highbeam.com/doc/IGI-112494569.html.

Who Is an Audiologist (AuD)? An Otolaryngologist (ENT)?

Let us begin by drawing a comparison that, while illustrative, may not be entirely fair: an audiologist is to an otorhinolaryngologist (or otolaryngologist), the ear, nose, and throat MD or DO (ENT), as an optometrist (OD) is to an ophthalmologist. Like ODs, audiologists are not MDs or DOs; however, a key difference from optometrists is that most do not claim to be.

Oto means ear, rhino means nose, larynx means back of the throat, and ology means rational study and knowledge.

The American Academy of Audiology states that audiologists are "primary healthcare professionals who evaluate, diagnose, treat, prevent, and manage hearing loss and balance disorders" in individuals of all ages. They program hearing aids, cochlear implants, assistive listening devices, bone-anchored hearing aids, and more.

Audiologists are more than just hearing instrument specialists, as some advertisements suggest; they also help diagnose deafness and other ear-related disorders. However, they are not the MDs or DOs who ultimately provide or confirm the final diagnosis or formulate treatment plans for most of these disorders.

ENTs are medical doctors (MDs or DOs) who specialize in disorders of the ear, nose, and throat, as well as the base of the skull and other areas of the head and neck. After completing their training in medical schools, they become the ones to perform corrective, reconstructive, and regional plastic surgery procedures.

An AuD candidate's education takes three to four years after obtaining a Bachelor of Science (BS) or Arts (BA) with a cumulative GPA of at least 2.75 to 3.0; this varies from school to school - and is not carried on at medical school.

AuD programs favor candidates who have completed undergraduate studies focused on audiology or have majored in sound engineering, communication disorders, language, or related fields, showcasing a genuine and lasting interest in the field.

The audiology degree is a doctoral degree, although it is not a medical one.

Adding both pre-graduate and graduate education, it takes about seven to eight years to earn an AuD at the doctoral level. The American Speech-Language-Hearing Association (ASHA) must approve an AuD graduate to be licensed or certified anywhere in the U.S. The ASHA certification provides definitive evidence of competence for direct clinical practice.

All that education is followed by licensing requirements in every state, usually through boards.

I have this concern: How can AuDs compete with TV advertisers for hearing aids under $250 and testing done through the telephone? I'll address that question in the latter chapters.

Despite all the AuD education and training, if someone suffers from auditory or balance disorders—issues that may arise from genetic or hereditary factors, autoimmune problems, brain or cerebellum tumors, inner ear diseases, hypertension, blood vessel inflammation, or medications, among other causes—the specialists to consult first, in my opinion, would be an ENT or ORL who are MDs or DOs. When referred by these doctors, patients should confidently go to an AuD.

References and Recommended Reading

1. "Become an Audiologist," The American Academy of Audiology, accessed on December 24, 2022, https://www.audiology.org/careers/become-an-audiologist.
2. Scott Wilson, "How to Become an Audiologist — Your Guide to Audiology Degree Requirements," SpeechPathologyGraduatePrograms.org, https;//www.speechpathologygraduateprograms.org/2021/09/become-an-audiologist.
3. "Otorhinolaryngology," Wikipedia, https://en.wikipedia.org/wiki/otorhinolaryngology.
4. "Pre-Audiology, BS," Stephen F. Austin University, https://catalog.sfasu.edu/preview_program.php?catoid=1&poid=287&returnto=26.
5. "What Is the Difference between Audiologists and ENT Doctors?" ENT Specialists, PC, https://omahaent.com/what-is-the-difference-between-audiologists-and-ent-doctors/.

Who Is a Physical Therapist (PT, DPT)? A Physiatrist?

Physical therapists (PTs) and doctors of physical therapy (DPTs) are healthcare professionals who develop and implement treatment plans prescribed by physiatrists and other medical providers seeking rehabilitation for their patients. This includes cardiologists, rheumatologists, orthopedic surgeons, neurologists, and various other physicians.

PTs work directly with patients of any age, from newborns to end-of-life patients, to help them maintain, improve, and restore physical movement affected by disease or injury. They assist in reducing or managing their pain.

PTs work in various settings, including outpatient clinics, rehabilitation facilities, hospitals, nursing homes, patients' homes, sports teams, and fitness centers. They help individuals achieve their fitness goals and regain active, independent living when it has been compromised.

While physical therapy was once a bachelor's degree and later a master's degree, it is now increasingly common for physical therapists (PTs) to obtain a Doctorate in Physical Therapy

(DPT). The American Physical Therapy Association expects all graduating PTs to hold a DPT degree by the end of this decade.

Still, this would not be comparable with an MD or DO degree.

Most DPT programs require at least three years of undergraduate education, but some accept students directly from high school into specific programs. No minimum GPA or MCAT score is necessary. The admission test used is the Graduate Record Examination (GRE®), which is a general test similar in format and content to the high school Standardized Admission Test (SAT).

PT graduate schools require an education in chemistry, biology, physics, exercise science, psychology, anatomy, and physiology as prerequisites for acceptance. According to the American Physical Therapy Association (APTA), the minimum GPA and GRE scores vary by institution.

DPT programs generally span three years. The first two years involve classroom instruction covering biology, anatomy, neurology, exercise physiology, biomechanics, clinical reasoning, evidence-based practice, communication, ethics, and values. Approximately 60–70 percent of this education occurs in the classroom, while the remainder comprises clinical experience. The final year of a DPT program usually includes hands-on clinical practice under the supervision of a licensed physical therapist.

After graduation, DPTs can pursue optional residencies and fellowships to advance the clinical practice of physical therapy while still receiving supervision and mentorship, or to deepen their expertise in a specific area.

DPTs can become board-certified specialists by meeting the requirements of the American Board of Physical Therapy Specialties (not a member of the ABMS nor the AOA) to prove greater depth of knowledge and clinical expertise in particular areas, including orthopedics, neurology, and geriatrics.

DPTs must obtain a state license to practice. As they are not MDs or DOs, they cannot prescribe medicines, but they may recommend over-the-counter medications.

Some PTs, like PAs and NPs, believe they can provide adequate patient care without referral or supervision. Therefore, they are now going to Congress to see if they can obtain this privilege. So, what's new?

A so-called "dangerous" bill that would have allowed DPTs direct access to patients without a referral was thwarted with bipartisan support a couple of years ago in the Texas House and Senate. However, they are at it again. Similar actions are occurring in other states—another never-ending story. So, what's new? (again).

PT primarily overlaps with chiropractic and physiatry. Physiatrists are either MDs or DOs and are the only professionals who can obtain board certification in physiatry or physical medicine and rehabilitation. Concerning the overlap with chiropractic, if you read the chapter on the latter, you know where I stand on the subject.

Physiatrists, or doctors of physical medicine and rehabilitation (PM&R), diagnose and treat patients with spinal cord injuries, sports injuries, and musculoskeletal and joint issues, such as back pain, arthritis, and fibromyalgia, as well as the consequences of brain trauma, strokes, and auto accidents.

Physiatrists, who are MDs or DOs in this field, can write prescriptions and administer various physical treatment modalities, including heat and cold therapy, infrared radiation, electrotherapy, massage, exercise, movement and activity modification, adaptive equipment, and orthotics such as braces, prostheses, exoskeletons, and similar devices.

Anyone requiring physical therapy should seek it from a PT; however, I prefer that this occurs only when a plan is prescribed and supervised by a physiatrist or another DO or MD. This professional should make the referral based on a proper diagnosis, recommend the treatment plan, and provide careful follow-up and collaboration.

References and Recommended Reading

1. "Becoming a Physical Therapist," American Physical Therapy Association, http://www.apta.org/AboutPTs/.
2. American Physical Therapy Association. *What Physical Therapists Do?* https://www.apta.org/your-career/careers-in-physical-therapy/becoming-a-pt
3. Fred Decker, "Physiatry vs. Physical Therapists," Chron, http://work.chron.com/physiatry-vs-physical-therapists-20460.html.
4. Casto, T. "How Did Medicine Fare in the Legislature?" *Dallas Med J.* 2015;101:199.
5. Commission on Accreditation in Physical Therapy Education, http://www.capteonline.org/home.aspx.

Who Is a Psychologist, a Psychotherapist, a Psychoanalyst, or a Psychiatrist?

Psychologists are professionals who study human behavior and practice mental health. They delve into "issues of the mind."

They evaluate and treat children and adults with mental, emotional, and social problems.

Prerequisites for entering psychology school vary; some will admit high school graduates, while others require a bachelor's degree with a GPA of around 2.5 or higher (in contrast to the GPA of around 4 for psychiatrists who must first be MDs or DOs) to progress to master's or doctoral programs in psychology.

While trying to understand the acronyms in this field, I encountered numerous terms used by psychologists—far too many to organize effectively. Therefore, I got creative and summarized them logically into:

1. Bachelor of Science or Arts in Psychology (PsyBS or PsyBA)
2. Master of Science or Arts in Psychology (PsyMS)

3. Doctor in Psychology (PsyD)
4. Doctor of Philosophy in Psychology (PsyPhD) (abbreviation of my creation for the lack of a straightforward or properly regulated one)

A bachelor's degree in psychology (level one) takes four years to complete and requires very little or no prior college education. Typically, it takes about six years to earn a master's degree (level two) and an additional one or two years to achieve a doctorate (levels three and four). An advanced degree is essential for working as a clinical or counseling psychologist, which can be either a PsyD (level three) or a PhD in psychology or sociology (level four).

Psychologists may specialize in research, counseling, school, industrial, and organizational psychology; however, the most common career path chosen by practitioners is clinical psychology.

A statistical analysis combining data from multiple studies (a meta-analysis) of the results of hundreds of publications by psychologists revealed that only a small percentage—about 5 percent- were reproducible. This is far too few for my comfort.

The above categorization leads us to the term "psychoanalyst," a branch of psychology traditionally linked to Sigmund Freud. Psychoanalysis, similar to "psychodynamic therapy," is a form of psychotherapy based on the idea that unconscious factors influence destructive behaviors and that recognizing these factors liberates patients from repetitive, disturbing, empty, or conflictual thoughts. Effectively addressing the causative factors, such as traumatic memories or stressors, enhances relationships with family, friends, and others.

Psychoanalysis may be a branch of psychology or psychiatry, but surprisingly, it does not require a degree in either field, as it is not a regulated term or profession.

To formally become a psychoanalyst, practitioners must complete an approved "intensive psychoanalytic training program" by the American Psychoanalytic Association (APsaA). To enter such a program, candidates should possess a bachelor's or graduate degree in a mental health-related field.

In some states, individuals may identify themselves as psychoanalysts, counselors, hypnotists, hypnotherapists, or psychotherapists without any verifiable formal education or training.

How can this possibly be?

Those titles, which are not adequately regulated, licensed, or controlled, allowing almost anyone to claim to be a psychoanalyst, open shop, and offer psychoanalytic services. Caveat emptor!

The field of medicine that overlaps most with psychology is psychiatry. A key difference between these two professions is that psychologists cannot prescribe medications, except in a limited number of states (five in 2020), while psychiatrists, being MDs or DOs, are permitted to prescribe FDA-approved medications.

Psychologists, even those with PhDs, do not attend MD or DO school. Therefore, they lack the authority to prescribe appropriate medications to patients with mental illnesses.

The process of qualifying for an ABMS or ABOM-recognized board certification in psychiatry can take twelve to fourteen years, involving rigorous exams throughout and at the conclusion of training.

Psychiatrists perform physical exams, order and interpret laboratory tests, order brain imaging studies such as MRI and CT scans, and prescribe psychotropic medications—the ones indicated to improve the mind, emotions, and behavior.

Psychiatrists can treat substance abuse, normalize intelligence deficits or surpluses, and address chronic anxiety, depression, bipolar behavior, and psychosis.

They can diagnose and manage brain tumors and metabolic diseases, such as metal poisoning (for example, mad hatter syndrome from mercury) and thyroid dysfunction, which may lead to behavioral disorders—even (vascular) blood vessel disorders like microembolisms that cause ministrokes. The University of Texas Tower shooter in 1966 serves as an example, as he had a brain tumor.

The belief that psychologists handle only minor mental issues while psychiatrists address major ones is incorrect. Such misconceptions can be harmful, primarily by delaying proper diagnosis and treatment.

Psychiatrists treat the full range of mental disorders, from mild to severe. They consider the patient's overall health in their clinical assessments and diagnoses. This allows them to prescribe medications while being mindful of potential drug interactions and side effects. Although psychiatrists can provide therapy, many focus primarily on medical management and collaborate with trusted psychologists for therapeutic support.

Meanwhile, as mentioned above, psychologists are skilled in various therapy techniques and can customize treatment plans to suit patients and their diagnoses. While psychologists receive training in psychotropic medications, they do not study the full range of health issues and drug interactions as extensively as psychiatrists do.

Beware of psychoanalysts without an MD or DO and of psychologists without a PsyD or PsyPhD suffix.

I often see oddball, uninformed individuals giving "expert opinions" on TV and other media, with titles below the presenters labeling them as "psychoanalysts," "psychotherapists," or occasionally even life coaches or influencers. How naive do they think their audience must be? I bet this happens because show producers and news anchors have yet to read this book or any relevant literature on the subject; therefore, they, too, are inadequately or improperly educated to determine whom to invite or have no idea what they are doing or worse, choose for ratings whoever may be available and willing.

In an article titled "Psychotherapy Reconsidered," the recently deceased Harriet Hall, MD (a.k.a. The SkepDoc), a highly regarded doctor, questions the effectiveness of psychotherapy (as I do) and its practitioners.

If it is indeed true that there are over six hundred modalities of psychotherapy, one advertisement on the radio, television, and social media informs listeners and viewers about a particular company they can call to connect clients in need with its 25,000 therapists. How can anyone not question the competence of the assigned therapist? It almost seems more plausible to think that such numbers pertain to the phone sex industry.

Incompetent practitioners, including skilled psychiatrists, have been known to inflict severe mental harm on clients—exacerbating depression, sexual dysfunction, and suicidal tendencies, for example. This is a delicate arena; therefore, mid-educated practitioners (MEPs) should not play with that fire.

It is my impression and recommendation that before consulting a psychotherapist, psychoanalyst, or even a psychologist with a PhD for mental health issues, one should first reach out to a psychiatrist (the only professional who can prescribe FDA-approved medications). Together, they can determine the best diagnosis, develop a treatment plan, and decide who will assist in carrying it out.

References and Recommended Reading

1. Kendra Cherry, "Can Psychologists Prescribe Medications?" Verywell Mind, May 5, 2020, https://www.verywellmind.com/can-psychologists-prescribe-medications-2795756.
2. Emily Decker, "Therapists Titles, or What do Those Letters After your Name Mean?" Medium.com, October 31, 2019, https://medium.com/@emely.jean.decker/therapist-titles-or-what-do-those-letter-after-your-name-mean-c109a0218ea.
3. "What Are the Education Requirements for Becoming a Psychologist?" Best Accredited Colleges, November 29, 2023, https://bestaccreditedcolleges.org/articles/education-need-to-become-a-psychologist.html.
4. Kathleen Curtis, "Step-by-Step Guide to Becoming a Psychologist," Student Training & Education in Public Service, https://www.publicservicedegrees.org/how-to-become/psychologist.
5. "How to Become a Licensed Clinical Psychologist," Study.com, http://education-portal.com//articles/How_toBecome_a_Licensed_Clinical_Psychologist_Career_Roadmap.html.
6. "Psychology or Psychiatry: Which Is Right for You?" WebMD, http://www.webmd.com/mental-health/features/psychology-vs-psychiatry-which -is-better.
7. "What Is Psychoanalysis?" Washington Center for Psychoanalysis, http://www.wcpweb.org/what-is-psychoanalysis.
8. American Psychoanalytic Association, www.apsa.org/.
9. Harriet Hall, "Psychotherapy Reconsidered," *Skeptic Magazine*, volume 28, 1, 2023.

What Is Complementary, Alternative, Integrative, and Functional Medicine?

The National Institutes of Health (NIH) has a division focused on Complementary and Alternative Medicine (CAM), known as the National Center for Complementary and Integrative Health (NCCIH), which was recently renamed the National Center for Complementary, Alternative, and Integrative Health (CAIH). The word "Medicine" was appropriately replaced with "Health," yet the name still feels far from ideal. CAIH encompasses a range of healthcare systems, practices, and products not typically recognized as part of conventional medicine, which I find to be of dubious value.

The changes in nomenclature prompt me to briefly discuss the meanings of the terms "complementary," "alternative," and "integrative, " first informing the reader that such language is constantly evolving.

- Complementary refers to a non-mainstream approach that is used alongside conventional medicine.
- Alternative refers to a non-mainstream approach used instead of conventional medicine.

- Integrative refers to coordinating conventional and complementary approaches by using them together.

Complementary approaches encompass tai chi, yoga, acupuncture, massage therapy, spinal manipulation, art therapy, music therapy, dance, mindfulness, chiropractic practices, osteopathic manipulations, including craniosacral therapy, meditation, relaxation techniques (such as breathing exercises), qigong, Rolfing, hypnotherapy, Reiki, and more. Additional practices include homeopathy, Ayurvedic medicine, traditional Chinese medicine, naturopathy, nutriology, and functional medicine. Practitioners are often referred to as "healers" or "teachers."

Many CAIH practitioners who identify as naturopaths or healers (terms I wish they wouldn't have misappropriated) peddle "natural" products, such as CBD in oil and other forms. "Natural" is a largely unregulated term. It encompasses botanicals or herbs, vitamins, amino acid peptides, particles, and minerals (sometimes marketed as colorful capsules or gummies that claim, without sufficient documentation from evidence-based medicine, to boost energy, aid weight loss, enhance happiness, improve clarity of thought, strengthen immunity, enhance sexual performance, and more), as well as pre-, pro-, and post-biotics; surely what used to be referred to as "snake oil." Don't forget that poison ivy, puffer fish, scorpion venom, snake venom, and cyanide, among others, are all "natural" products that can be harmful and even lethal.

Some CAIH practitioners may perform chiropractic adjustments, massage therapies, "healing" touches, nearly touching, reflexology, acupressure, transcendental meditation, biofeedback, cupping, colonic cleansing, chelation, and more. Ugh!

As a taxpayer, you should know that the National Institutes of Health (NIH) has an annual operational cost of over $50 billion. Of this amount, the NCCIH consumed nearly $160 million in 2021 and requested a budget exceeding $184 million for 2022. Remember, this organization is accused of financing, at least in part, research in China linked to the development of the virus that caused the COVID-19 epidemic. In this era of cost containment, I would advocate closing or defunding the NCCIH.

Congress established the Office of Complementary, Alternative, and Integrative Health to define, through rigorous scientific investigation, the effectiveness and safety of complementary and integrative health interventions and their roles in enhancing health and healthcare.

According to my calculations, over the past ten years (with annual budgets averaging $130 to $160 million), the NCCIH (including the period when it was known as NCCAM) consumed nearly $1.5 billion. Uff!

What for?

The NCCIH has been criticized for funding and marketing pseudoscientific medicine.

It discovered that meditation and mindfulness may help with anxiety and depression, reduce insomnia, alleviate symptoms of post-traumatic stress disorder (PTSD), assist in recovery from substance abuse, support weight loss efforts, improve eating behaviors, and enhance the immune function marker (IL-6) in lonely older adults. At the same time, some individuals might experience negative outcomes. (Lots of "mays," huh?)

This, to me, represents money wasted on a bunch of nonsense. But then again, I thought the same about the effects of cow farting studies on the ozone hole.

The NCCIH identified an association between chronic severe back pain and certain disabilities through a national survey. Remarkably, it also found out that yogic breathing may influence the flow of the fluid surrounding the spine without speculating on how this would benefit any specific human disease. Another finding is that yoga and physical therapy (PT) may improve lower back pain, although not significantly. (Did you catch the sarcasm?)

Moreover, there are very few other expensive discoveries of this nature. Most negate the value of CAIH. They are, instead, self-defeating propositions that should lead to the agency's closure.

Every day, people still consult CAIH practitioners and spend, if not waste, tens of billions of dollars on office visits and "medicines" that don't work and can be purchased over the counter (OTC) without a prescription, which is all that these practitioners are allowed to recommend.

A 2016 National Center for Health Statistics study reported that a substantial number of Americans spend an average of $500 annually on non-covered, non-reimbursable CAIH. This should alert conventional medicine doctors that we must do better, such as educating patients and properly marketing ourselves, the latter of which I would loathe to do.

In 2012, Americans spent $3 billion just on homeopathy, a form of CAIH, out of the $34 billion spent on alternative medicine (adjust that for inflation over the past decade). That year, the Australian government examined all available evidence on homeopathy. In 2015, it concluded that "Americans are wasting their money." To that, the Aussies added that homeopathy "should not be used to treat health conditions that are chronic, serious, or could become serious."

Please understand, as I mentioned earlier, that what is often referred to as "mainstream medicine" or, as CAIH practitioners prefer to label it in a derogatory manner, "allopathic medicine," would gladly welcome and integrate any treatment proven to be effective in the realm of alternative medicine. Once termed "heroic," allopathy has evolved into evidence-based medicine (EBM).

For example, and not that I agree with it, some "allopaths" or mainstream doctors have recommended St. John's Wort for mild depression, even while aware of its potential for severe drug-to-drug interactions. Some orthopedic surgeons suggest chondroitin and turmeric capsules for "bone-to-bone" osteoarthritis. A psychiatrist friend who took turmeric developed a severe blood disorder that resulted in passing clots in his urine, which supports my skepticism about the safety of botanicals as portrayed in TV ads. Some family physicians advise insomniacs to take melatonin, and some cardiologists recommend omega-3 oils from fish or krill for their patients. I want to emphasize that we allopaths are not opposed to botanicals, provided adequate proof of their efficacy and safety exists in evidence-based medicine. All this I said to tell you not to be gullible and to question much of what one sees advertised, particularly on television.

Let me now share a couple of personal anecdotes, although I would prefer not to, as I advise against believing anecdotes; I will also include some public-domain examples related to CAIH and functional medicine.

The wife of one of my patients was informed by oncologists from two highly reputable medical centers that she had pancreatic cancer for which reasonable treatment options were unavailable (the prognosis for this type of cancer has improved in recent years). The husband took her to an alternative medicine clinic in Tijuana, Mexico, where she soon passed away. My patient was told that this happened because they wasted critical time while under the care of American doctors.

Steve McQueen went to a renowned clinic in Rosarito Beach, Mexico, for lung cancer that U.S. doctors deemed incurable. There, he received treatments involving pancreatic enzymes and about fifty pills a day, primarily vitamins and minerals, along with massages, prayers, coffee enemas, injections of sheep and cattle fetal extracts, and Laetrile® (a medication also known as amygdalin)—a substance derived from apricot pits that has side effects similar to those of cyanide, to which it converts in the body, and for which no evidence-based medicine supports its effectiveness. Laetrile's popularity, now dwindling, stemmed from many anecdotal reports. Tragically, McQueen died four months after his arrival, suffering from widespread metastasis.

Both understandably turned to CAIH since conventional medicine could not cure them.

My peeve is never with the patients, of course, but with those who consciously exploit the desperate and vulnerable. The patient's husband believed what CAIH practitioners told him instead of mainstream doctors. Such is the manipulative power of quackery and its marketing. My patient ended up a widower, sad, angry, and devastated.

Although stories like these are often heard, patients continue to flock to, consult with, and receive incompetent (mind you) treatment from CAIH practitioners until they become disenchanted with them—and, sadly and unfairly, with medicine in general.

It is possible that we, as mainstream doctors, carry much of the blame for not setting proper expectations, giving insufficient time to adequately inform our patients, not allowing them to express their concerns during seemingly brief office visits, demonstrating poor bedside manners, or simply failing them without a credible explanation.

Even the best medicine, provided by the finest doctors in the most advanced facilities, cannot cure everyone. Doctors who experience failure are not always to blame; they also endure pain and suffering when they are unable to heal or save lives.

It is common for patients, even with the best intentions, to begin with unrealistic expectations, misguided beliefs, uneducated philosophies about health, improper attitudes, or incorrect values and priorities. They and we need to address this during our encounters.

Patients whom MDs or DOs cannot cure are likely to suffer again in their bodies and souls, especially when CAIH lets them down. This is particularly true when their finances are impacted. CAIH services are generally not covered by insurance or other third-party payors. Some exceptions exist, notably chiropractic care, which Veterans Affairs covers, and some insurance plans do as well. Additionally, certain states mandate insurance companies to reimburse for naturopathy. In my view, this represents a misappropriation of funds.

CAIH practitioners rarely receive meaningful medical training beyond high school or college, and their schools do not provide any. Furthermore, they typically lack direct access to diagnostic tools such as X-rays, EKGs, laboratories, and other equipment essential for accurate diagnosis and effective treatment planning.

Due to these limitations, CAIH providers must, and typically do, rely on the diagnoses provided by their patients that were confirmed by actual medical doctors. However, they often project an air of (false) competence in managing their clients' conditions.

Much of the illness that quacks treat tends to be self-limited and non-life-threatening. Otherwise, they wouldn't "look good" if one of their patients worsens, dies, or reads this book. Notice that they primarily focus on aches, acne, allergies, digestive issues, depression, fibromyalgia, and conditions that allow them to profit without risking their reputation, which is already on a tightrope, while disregarding the actual health and quality of their clients.

I contend that CAIH is largely a waste of time, hope, and money that would be better invested in mainstream (allopathic) medical care and that neither private nor government insurers should cover it.

Understand that "integrative" is merely a rebranding, likely for marketing purposes or an attempt to obscure the poor reputation of "alternative" and "complementary" medicine. Additionally, I find the use of "integrative" by CAIH practitioners disrespectful to mainstream medical doctors, as it suggests that MDs or DOs are hesitant to treat patients in a "wholistic" or "holistic" ("body as a whole") manner, which is generally not true.

The following are some forms of CAIH that I liken to quackery:

Homeopathy

Homeopathy is a type of CAIH approach to health care that, as stated in a current webpage of the NIH, is "based on the belief that natural substances, prepared in a very unique and peculiar way, to be used most often in tiny amounts, would restore health."

For homeopaths, a remedy is considered effective if it causes a healthy person to experience the same symptoms as those of an ill patient. This, they claim, would "induce the body to heal itself."

However, a 2010 report from the House of Commons Science and Technology Committee of the United Kingdom

(UK) states that the highly diluted substances they recommend "perform no better than placebo (dummy treatments)."

In 2017, the National Health Service (NHS) of England-UK declared that "homeopathic remedies will no longer be available on prescription" because it is a misuse of funds. Specifically, the NHS qualifies homeopathy as a poor replacement for available medical treatments that have their value based on scientific evidence, saying it is "at complete odds with our modern understanding of biology, chemistry, and physics."

Mainstream medicine uses terms such as "pseudoscience," "sham," and "quackery" to describe homeopathy.

Only a few of the numerous studies support the efficacy of homeopathic medications; most equate their effectiveness to that of a placebo ("sugar pills").

Examples of homeopathic remedies include ipecac (a vomitive), prescribed by homeopaths to treat vomiting; highly diluted red onion, used for treating conjunctivitis (as it causes eyes to become red and watery); and pollen, utilized to manage allergies. Preparations made from poison ivy, arsenic, crushed bees, and arnica also exist; you figure out what they might be used for.

Homeopathic medications can be dangerous, either due to severe reactions to their ingredients or indirectly, by postponing the prescription of suitable medications by allopathic practitioners who adhere to evidence-based medicine (EBM).

In 2023, the credible magazine *Skeptical Inquirer* questioned a publication on homeopathy for lung cancer, which showed surprisingly good benefits. The magazine concluded that the data could only be explained by "manipulation or falsification." Replies are under review at the time of this writing. The report illustrates the potential "fake news" one confronts when interpreting homeopathic literature. My take is that it's best not to trust it.

A tutorial explaining how to prepare homeopathic remedies has become available on the internet; it (accidentally?) illustrates that many such medicaments may contain only diluents like water and alcohol. This supports the claims of homeopathy critics who argue that if remedies are diluted to their twelve centesimal potencies (a typical dilution noted as "12C" or "24X" on the label), their "working" (the term "active" cannot be declared) ingredient becomes virtually undetectable, as not even one molecule would remain. This would explain not only their inefficacy but also their purported safety.

Some homeopaths go as far as to attribute the effectiveness of their preparations to a sort of "memory" of the "active" ingredient remaining in its diluents, like water or flavored syrup.

While rare, homeopathic products can cause adverse events and undesirable interactions with beneficial medications that the patient may be using for other conditions. Therefore, they can also be harmful on their own. Always read the labels!

Although the Food and Drug Administration (FDA) regulates the manufacturing processes and other standards for homeopathic drugs to ensure compliance with purity, strength, and quality, it does not regulate their effectiveness.

The Center for Inquiry's Office of Public Policy in DC recently recommended that the agency implement strict guidelines requiring homeopathic products to meet the same standards as nonhomeopathic drugs.

No homeopathic products are "approved" by the FDA to medicate patients. Be aware that some homeopathic "medicaments" are sold at pharmacy chains, possibly fraudulently displayed alongside truly effective medications. Remember, read the labels!

Some homeopathic products can be sold over-the-counter (OTC) because they are intended to treat minor, self-limited conditions that the consumer can self-diagnose. Even if they may be ineffective, as long as they are not harmful, buyer beware!

Homeopathic drugs intended to treat serious health conditions can only be prescribed by licensed medical practitioners, such as MDs or DOs who have become homeopaths, and there are some. What a waste of education! I say.

Homeopaths explain and argue that because homeopathic treatments are tailored to each individual rather than solely focusing on their illnesses, patients with the same diagnosis may receive completely different homeopathic formulations. I wish to emphasize that those treatments are based on findings of doubtful validity and the personal or anecdotal experience of the homeopath, not on EBM.

There are no national or international standards for training homeopathy practitioners. As a licensed medical doctor, I could take a few courses, some of which might only be a weekend long, or read texts about the subject on my own, and then hang a shingle in front of my office and call myself a homeopath because the title is so poorly regulated. Aspiring homeopaths may study at a certifying organization, learn the trade from established homeopaths, take online classes, or do some home studying from textbooks one could buy at Barnes & Noble or Amazon.

No diploma or certificate from any medical school licenses providers to practice homeopathy in the U.S. Some states allow MDs or DOs to engage in this practice. Homeopathy is not officially recognized as a healthcare method nationwide, nor are there any board certifications accepted by the ABMS or AOA.

In an effort to keep an open mind, I listened to homeopaths at several medical meetings to ensure I wasn't depriving my patients of anything, especially those who were not responding to my treatments. However, the lectures contributed nothing of value, reinforcing my belief that homeopathy and its remedies are a waste of time, money, and hope.

Worse yet, regarding coverage, people with limited incomes should be made aware that Medicare or Medicaid will likely not cover homeopathy, which is unavailable on Parts A and B.

I recommend, as the British and Australian governments do, that homeopathy be dismissed altogether as a form of health care, at least to my readers.

Hormesis

I briefly touch on this to dispel the notion that hormesis is a form or subset of homeopathy; it is not.

It investigates drugs that have varying effects depending on the dose, such as inhibitory effects at low doses and stimulatory effects at high doses. The implication is that the same substance, which can be toxic at moderate to high doses, may be beneficial at low doses; for instance, alcohol can be lethal in high doses but relaxing in low doses. For example, low-calorie diets may aid in weight loss, potentially extending lifespan, while high-calorie diets can lead to weight gain and a shortened life. Minor stressors on brain neurons or muscles might promote longevity, but major stressors can be fatal. Substances that are toxic in higher doses but probably beneficial in lower ones include selenium, iron, zinc, glutamic acid, arsenic, resveratrol (found in wine and grape juice—though this is debatable), sulforaphane (present in broccoli), capsaicin (found in jalapeños), and curcumin (derived from Indian saffron). Metformin, a medicine for Type 2 diabetes, increases the uptake of insulin by some tissues, lowering glucose and HbA1c. Some antidepressants block serotonin reuptake; they conceivably work through hormesis.

The only similarities between hormesis and homeopathy are the "ho" and that both try remedies in low doses. Hormesis is in its infancy; take it with a grain of salt.

Herbalism

Also referred to as "herbal medicine," herbalism should have gone the way of leeches at barbershops or, better yet, the dodo bird. (I feel more pity for dodos than for herbalists prescribing botanicals.)

I acknowledge that excellent medications originate from botanical sources, including digoxin, a heart failure medication; curarine, a muscle relaxant used in anesthesia; vincristine, an agent for cancer chemotherapy; and various antibiotics and immune modulators that prevent the rejection of transplanted organs. These are FDA-regulated, and their preparations are standardized; therefore, they differ from the herbal concoctions sold without proper regulation.

I remind those who choose medications or treatments because they are regarded as "natural" that poison ivy, cyanide, scorpion and snake venoms, bee sting allergens, hallucinogenic mushrooms, and many other substances also have natural origins.

Hundreds of reports have been published regarding the toxicities linked to herbal medicines. You can search for them on Google or find them at FDA.gov.

A selection of Chinese herbs was recently reported to have caused an epidemic of irreversible kidney damage, necessitating lifelong dialysis or transplantation.

Some products have been found to contain hidden ingredients, as was the case with ephedra, which led to deaths from heart damage. Licorice is known to trigger hypertensive crises (high blood pressure), deplete potassium, and potentially cause brain damage or death. The root of black cohosh, which belongs to the buttercup family and is sold to alleviate menopausal symptoms, resulted in liver failures that necessitated transplantation before being recalled. A zinc formulation for the topical treatment of psoriasis was pulled from the market because it contained undisclosed steroids that caused weight gain and stretch marks in children.

Be aware that the limited way the government regulates herbal and natural medicines only serves to prevent their marketers from making medical claims. These products must be labeled as "dietary supplements" and cannot claim to be "safe and effective" but merely "safe," if at all. Many products, once proven harmful or deadly, are banned. But that may happen when it's too late.

One advantage of herbal products is that they are generally inexpensive, making them more accessible to populations that cannot afford certain prescription drugs (an issue for my next book).

It is indisputable that many branded pharmaceuticals are absurdly expensive, causing a significant portion of the United States population to be priced out of them. I observe this in my daily practice and attribute it to a multitude of factors, not merely, as many think, the pharmaceutical companies.

In the three months leading up to the completion of my reviews for this chapter, the FDA and FTC published approximately seventy-five alerts and advisories regarding herbal products. These included recalls for undeclared ingredients, false claims, and scams. Notably, many weight loss products, beauty items, juices or extracts from cacti and ginseng, products for joint pain and swelling, as well as herbal Viagra." I cannot help but mention some product names like Black Mamba Premium by SX Power Co, African Superman by R. Thomas Marketing, and Bigger Longer More Sperms at biggerlongermorsperms.com (not kidding). Guess what they suggest? I am laughing too hard while typing this.

I advise avoiding herbalists and their products, at least until both become regulated.

Anyone considering an herbal remedy should carefully weigh the associated risks and consult an MD or DO instead of a naturopathic or functional physician, particularly if there may be a financial interest. These risks may not be fully disclosed and could be significant. For instance, the once-popular St. John's Wort, which is used to treat mild depression (without strong support from EBM), can cause rashes, sexual dysfunction, fatigue, gastrointestinal upset, confusion, rapid heartbeat, and high blood pressure. It may also interact harmfully with SSRIs and MAOIs, both of which are also used for depression, as well as some antipsychotics, birth control pills, several blood thinners, immune modulators for organ rejection, and more.

For any herbal product you may be taking or may wish to take, check for drug interactions, not just for the validity of their use.

The key takeaway is to be cautious of advertisements and promotions for herbal remedies, which are abundant on television and radio.

Don't trust the half-truths (equivalent to half-lies) presented in hour-long infomercials, which are often aired after midnight or on purchased time, including social media platforms that feature "doctors" of the kind I have repeatedly exposed as quacks and crooks. For your safety's sake, avoid buying and taking herbal medications and unproven supplements. Steer clear of them.

Chelation

This term refers to a chemical reaction in which a specific bond forms a molecule known as a "chelate." Agents that facilitate such bonds are referred to as chelators. The resulting molecule may sequester a specific chemical that could be implicated in a medical issue—in ways that may or may not be beneficial.

Conventional medicine employs chelators to treat poisoning from metals such as mercury, lead, arsenic, copper, and even iron, which can accumulate in the body under certain situations (such as lead exposure in children who have licked paint or iron and copper accumulation in certain liver diseases). However, chelation is also advocated in CAIH to address conditions for which there is no substantial evidence of its efficacy.

The American Medical Association (AMA), the American Heart Association (AHA), the American Cancer Society (ACS), the FDA, and the NIH have all clearly indicated, in one form or another, that there is no adequate, well-controlled published data (EBM) to support the use of chelation in cardiovascular disease or cancer, which is widely promoted by quacks.

A well-known example of chelation misuse is its association with autism. For decades, autism was wrongly blamed on thimerosal, a mercury-based preservative previously used in some vaccines. The author who popularized this claim was ultimately exposed as a fraud and had his medical license revoked in the UK, where he practiced. However, the damage had already been done. Since the revelation of this falsehood, the use of chelation for autism has diminished significantly.

Chelation therapy may lead to liver and kidney damage, cardiac arrhythmias, and even death.

Studies aimed at supporting chelation have faced criticism from respected medical organizations as "unethical," "risky," "pointless," and "wasteful" in reputable medical journals. Systematic reviews indicate that chelation is no more effective than a placebo and can sometimes be dangerous.

I recommend avoiding chelation therapy practitioners unless an MD or DO prescribes it for an approved indication, such as metal poisoning. Additionally, chelation therapy should be conducted at a reputable hospital or clinic that is equipped to monitor and manage potential complications.

Colonics

Colon cleansing through oral powders, liquid laxatives, enemas, or irrigations is one of the most ridiculous rituals a person can subject themselves to, as if they are unclean internally.

Even if performed to alleviate fatigue, boost immunity, treat acne, reduce skin wrinkles, combat foul body odor, manage arthritis, address menstrual irregularities, improve liver function, relieve constipation, tackle diarrhea, curb food cravings, ease indigestion, eliminate halitosis, reduce burping, minimize flatulence, address malabsorption, and assist with obesity-related conditions for which it is claimed to be effective, I would not recommend a colonic to anyone.

Some CAIH practitioners even prescribe colonics for inflammatory bowel disease (IBD) and diverticular disease (which can easily become inflamed and perforate), for which they are likely contraindicated.

The practice of colonic hydrotherapy is based on two bizarre and absurd premises:

1. The colon allows some "toxins" within it to escape into the circulation and be sent to the skin (imagine the stench), the lungs (imagine the halitosis), the brain (imagine the "fog"), and other organs where they would cause harm, like wrinkles and depression.

   Some practitioners exploit the so-called "leaky gut syndrome" for their convenience. In this condition, the normal protective bacterial levels in the intestine may be disrupted, potentially allowing for the passage of immune reaction triggers, leading to inflammation and accounting for various illnesses, such as lupus or the spread of melanomas. Colonics may exacerbate the condition for which they were performed.

2. Inserting a pipe or tube into one's anus and then up the rectum and colon (good luck finding a more elegant language) to rinse them with water or saline solutions (sometimes enhanced with herbs, coffee, or other substances) purifies and detoxifies the entire body.

Problems with colonics are twofold:

1. There are no adequately conducted and validated studies to support most of the claims made by its practitioners.
2. There is significant potential for harm and even death. Heart and liver failure, electrolyte imbalances, intestinal perforation from incorrect prodding with irrigation tubes, hemorrhoidal bleeding, ruptured diverticula or inflamed colon walls, and the spreading of infections including hepatitis and amoebiasis (an intestinal parasitosis with dysentery—google it) have all been reported.

Although the FDA does not regulate the colonics industry (which I believe it should—or someone should), it has repeatedly warned suppliers about misleading claims of effectiveness, safety concerns, and quality-control violations.

Unless in oral preparation prior to a colonoscopy, as prescribed and performed by a qualified gastroenterologist, I would suggest avoiding colonics. They are ineffective for nearly everyone.

Reiki

This is a holistic Japanese technique for spiritual healing. "Rei" refers to higher knowledge, while "Ki" signifies life energy. Touted for its ability to produce "miraculous cures, relieve pain, assist with emotional and coping issues, and ease the transition to death," this "healing" invokes an "energy style of medical treatment" where energy is channeled from a practitioner's hands, placed on or near the recipient. Sometimes, this is applied over an injury to activate or enhance a "natural and inherently intelligent healing energy."

No EBM data supports it, and there is no evidence that such "energy" exists. If you're craving something Japanese, I recommend tempura.

Forget any photographic trickery associated with the so-called "auras" surrounding the body. These claims have been thoroughly debated and debunked in skeptical publications.

Reiki has neither been shown to be harmful nor helpful. But it should not delay, much less replace, conventional medical care, even when much human disease is self-limited.

Money or the hope needed for medical care should not be invested or wasted in this form of CAIH.

Rolfing

This type of therapy is named after its creator, Ida Rolf, an alternative medicine practitioner. A biochemist, Dr. Rolf proposed that external factors misalign the "integration of self with gravity" and that working on fascia (the tissue covering muscles) could alleviate stress.

No quality scientific literature has been produced to validate such a bizarre claim. Rolfing may be nothing more than a glorified form of massage.

Again, like with Reiki, I advise against spending (or wasting) money or hope on this form of CAIH.

Acupuncture

In its original form, as practiced in traditional Chinese medicine, acupuncture involves inserting thin needles through the skin into specific points on the body. This practice enables Qi (a form of "vital healing energy") to flow through channels within the body called meridians.

Acupuncture is intended to correct imbalances in the flow of Qi that lead to pain and various medical conditions.

EBM does not support the claims of benefits from acupuncture beyond placebo effects. However, it allows for its use in treating a few conditions, such as chronic lower back pain, certain allergies, and specific types of headaches.

Although complications are rarely reported, including lung punctures, infections, and death, most are attributed to operator inexperience and incompetence.

Acupuncture is widely practiced in China. In Texas, where I run my practice, it is regulated by the State Board of Medicine.

Acupuncture is questionable and, in my view, a last-resort adjunct for treating certain painful conditions that have not responded solely to conventional medicine.

In the words of Edzard Ernst, MD, emeritus professor at the University of Exeter, UK, and formerly an alternative healthcare practitioner, "Providing good care with empathy and compassion could be much more effective and less expensive than acupuncture." Dr. Ernst supports his assertion with thorough statistical analyses and data that are quite difficult to dispute.

Acupressure

This is one of many variants of acupuncture; it applies pressure with fingers, heat, or lasers instead of needles (to not discourage those who are needle-phobic) without evidence of superiority compared to the (placebo?) effects of conventional acupuncture, and it may reduce its risks and complications.

Reflexology

This "healing art" operates on the premise that glands and organs within the body have corresponding areas located primarily on the feet, as well as on the hands and ears. When these areas are pressed, the function of the represented organ or gland improves.

Reflexology is said to work by unblocking the healing energy, known as Qi, which we mentioned in our discussion on acupuncture. This practice allegedly "balances" the nervous system and releases chemicals to alleviate stress and pain.

Once again, there is no scientifically valid evidence for the existence of Qi or that the healing claimed to result from unblocking Qi actually takes place. Reflexology is another example of "so-called alternative medicine (SCAM)." Oh, what a delightful acronym.

Iridology

This pseudoscience examines the iris to offer a diagnosis and guide treatment.

It is based on the obviously ridiculously flawed assumption that each body part has representation in the iris, similar to how reflexology is said to work on the ears, hands, or feet. Iridologists examine the eye, particularly the iris, and claim to discern whether an internal organ or gland is healthy without needing to test or examine those organs more directly and thoroughly.

In conventional medical practice, features of high cholesterol, iron, or copper excess and deposition can be identified along the iris margins; however, this is not the essence of iridology.

Plenty of studies have proven iridology to be another baseless and useless SCAM.

Cupping

This is based on the hypothesis that practitioners can extract through the skin the causes of pain, swelling, muscle knots, colds, bronchitis, pneumonia, arthritis, infertility, and even some blood disorders where common medical sense finds it contraindicated.

Negative pressure inside cups, balls, bells, cow horns, bamboo stalks, and more- created by heating the air within these devices while attached to the skin- is believed to remove harmful miasmas (unhealthy odors or vapors emanating from ill bodies).

Suction cups made of neoprene may gain popularity as they use sophisticated motorized pumps for suctioning, making the procedure feel high-tech and cool.

You may have seen swimmers competing in the Olympics and basketball players with circular bruises from cupping. I have been consulted for severe bruising in patients with platelet disorders, even those induced by aspirin, where the lesions took on grotesque appearances. Search for examples on Google, and you'll understand what I mean; you will be horrified.

I find cupping to be another SCAM, a form of faith healing that does not work and causes adverse sequelae.

Hypnosis and Hypnotherapy

I tested the waters of hypnosis for a while, sometimes seemingly successfully. I left it because EBM poorly supports it. Maybe I lacked the patience and time to perform it correctly, but I think it works.

Hypnosis relies on the power of suggestion. Inducing altered states of consciousness, often referred to as "trances," enables some individuals to voluntarily submit, albeit temporarily, to the guidance of a hypnotist.

Hypnotherapy involves using hypnosis to help recover suppressed memories and modify behaviors, such as overeating, smoking, or vomiting. While its success is limited, it is not negligible. Serious hypnotherapy differs significantly from the hypnosis presented for theatrical purposes.

If someone plans to agree to hypnotherapy, I suggest that it be performed by psychiatrists or their recommended and supervised professional.

Functional Medicine

A more accurate term for this practice might be dysfunctional medicine, as it stems from both the patient and the provider experiencing some form of brain dysfunction. However, that is just my opinion.

Periodically, patients come into my office and tell me their "doctor" is a functional medicine specialist. I immediately know that what follows will be harrowing for me. Those patients have been fed beliefs (brain cockroaches, I call them) that are difficult to reverse, fumigate, and eliminate.

Typically, these patients present extensive lists of irrelevant lab results, often including cortisol levels, various metals, and rare earth elements, displayed on professional-looking, multicolored sheets of paper. To me, this implies that the clinical laboratory that performed these tests is involved in the SCAM.

While searching PubMed™, the most reliable and comprehensive source of medical information from the NIH (often referred to as a sort of medical Google), many publications that collate "Medicine and Function" mislead searchers by inadequately integrating the two terms (over three million in total). Therefore, I will paraphrase Wikipedia for you: Functional medicine is an alternative form of health care that includes unproven and disproven treatments based on interactions between the environment and the body, including its digestive tract, endocrine system, and immune systems, to create individualized therapies.

Functional medicine, another rebranded form of CAIH, has been labeled "pseudoscientific" and "quackery," even though some prestigious schools offer education on the topic (in my opinion, to their discredit).

Training somebody as a functional medicine provider takes as little as ten months of online studies, potentially less, as there is no recognized standard for it. Compare that to the twelve years it takes to train a specialized MD or DO. Ridiculous!

Miscellaneous

Music therapy, cosmetic procedures (ranging from shaving to applying makeup for hospitalized patients), humor, dog visits, nutritional guidance, and similar approaches are likely to yield benefits, such as reduced pain and shorter hospital stays. These enhancements are all welcomed and appreciated by those who are unwell. Even when they may not provide direct benefits, these therapies are not criticized here, as they are harmless and can offer distraction and happiness to patients.

I conclude this chapter by insisting that my readers be wary of the CAIH practitioners and quacks out there who are after their money.

I find it amazing that there are human beings like the CAIH practitioners who believe, in their "heart of hearts" (whatever that is), that they are accurately diagnosing patients by examining irises, for example, or properly treating the very sick by rechanneling their negative energies, pulling miasmas out of bodies into cups, and more, without feeling guilty for at least delaying proper medical care from evidence-based medicine provided by real doctors. They do not realize that what they (CAIH, functional medicine practitioners, and other quacks) are doing is laughing, on their way to the bank, at vulnerable, sick people who deserve better.

Ask anyone who practices SCAM whether they would go to another CAIH provider if they developed low PaO2 (oxygen pressure in the blood) in the context of COVID-19 or exhibited symptoms and signs of a stroke, heart attack, or metastatic melanoma. I bet they won't.

References and Recommended Reading

1. David Brown, "Scientists Speak Out Against Federal Funds for Research on Alternative Medicine," *The Washington Post*, March 17, 2009. ISSN 0190-8286.
2. Ernst Edzard, "No Alternative," New Scientist, April 26, 2008.
3. "Complementary, Alternative, or Integrative Health: What's in a Name?" National Center for Complementary and Integrative Health, US Department of Health and Human Services, accessed on December 3, 2022, https://www.nccih.nih.gov/health/complementary-alternative-or-integrative-health-whats-in-a-name.
4. Belluz J. *Vox*. 11 Mar 2015. Emory S. Homeopathy Doesn't Work. So Why Do So Many Germans Believe in It? *Bloomberg Business Week*. 12 Oct. 2021.
5. Barron H. Lerner, "McQueen's Legacy of Laetrile," *The New York Times*, November 15, 2005, www.nytimes.com/2005/11/15/health/15essa.html.
6. Liz Szabo, "Alternative Therapies and Supplements Can Cause Side Effects," *USA Today*, June 18, 2013, https://www.usatoday.com/story/news/nation/2013/06/18/alternative-therapies-supplements-effectiveness/2429465/.
7. Homeopathy Plus!, www.homeopathyplus.com.au.
8. David Gorski, "A Truly Homeopathic Defense of Homeopathy, Science-Based Medicine, December 17, 2012, www.sciencebasedmedicine.org/homeopathy-as-nanoparticles/.

9. The US Food and Drug Administration, www.fda.gov.
10. The American Institute of Homeopathy, www.homeopathyusa.org.
11. Homeopathic Directory, www.homeopathicdirectory.com.
12. Jeff Dellinger, "Homeopathy on Trial: CFI Suits against Walmart and CVS on Consumer Fraud Allowed to Proceed," *Skeptical Inquirer*, January/February 2023, p. 7.
13. Menachem Oberbaum, Shepherd Roee Singer, and Noah Samuels, "Hormesis and Homeopathy: Bridge over Troubled Waters," *Human & Experimental Toxicology*, 2010;29:567–571.
14. "Hormesis," Wikipedia, http://en.wikipedia.org/wiki/Hormesis.
15. Myers, J. P., "Hormesis Is a Flawed Theory," http://www.ourstolenfuture.org/Commentary/JPM/2006-1005hormesisflawed.html.
16. Frazier, K, "CFI Testimony Urges FDA to Regulate Homeopathic Products," Skeptical inquirer, 2015;39:6–7.
17. Michael F. Picco, "Can Colon Cleansing Get Rid of Toxins from the Body?" Mayo Clinic, http://mayoclinic.org/healthy-living/consumer-health/expert-answers/colon-cleansing/faq-20058435.
18. Nashville Reiki, http://reikinashvilletn.com.
19. M. S. Lee, M. H. Pittler, and E. Ernst, "Effects of Reiki in Clinical Practice: A Systematic Review of Randomized Clinical Trials," *International Journal of Clinical Practice*, 2008:62:947–954.
20. E. Ernst, "Applying Science to SCAM: A Brief Summary of the Past Thirty Years," *Skeptical Inquirer*, January/February 2022, pp. 11–12.
21. Norbert Aust and Viktor Weisshäupl, "Homeopathy Hits a New Low," *Skeptical Inquirer*, May–June 2023, pp. 41–8.

Who Is a Naturopathic Physician, Doctor, or Naturopath (ND, NMD)?

Naturopathic medicine is a type of CAIH that relies on natural therapies and the body's ability to stay healthy or heal itself. It is practiced by naturopathic physicians or "doctors" (NDs). They can hold either a "doctorate of naturopathy" (ND) or a "doctorate of naturopathic medicine" (NMD). The only difference between these degrees lies in their titles.

To clarify from the outset, no medical schools that confer MD or DO degrees offer programs for ND or NMD degrees; naturopaths attend institutions that only teach naturopathy.

In most states, NDs and NMDs cannot prescribe FDA-approved medications. Furthermore, naturopathy is entirely prohibited in several states.

NDs and NMDs provide nutritional recommendations, botanical products such as herbs, homeopathy, psychological guidance, counseling, and a variety of addendums, all of which are poorly, if at all, supported by EBM.

Naturopathy posits that modern medications should be avoided in favor of entirely natural products. The use of prescription medications stands in stark contrast to naturopathy, which benefits practitioners since they are rarely permitted to prescribe medications.

Other recommendations they make include colonics, iridology, hydrotherapy, reflexology, detoxifying soles, and abstaining from alcohol and sugar. They criticize certain medicines and foods as being "bad for you," while suggesting alternatives such as meditation, Rolfing, Reiki, brainwave entrainment, chelation, traditional Chinese and Indian medicine, lifestyle counseling, and other forms of CAIH.

Notice that at the end of advertisements for naturopathic products attempting to assert medical benefits, it states in tiny and blurry print that the FDA has not approved them. ("Certified" does not equate to "approved." Remember?)

According to an organization known as the Association of Accredited Naturopathic Medical Colleges and the Council on Naturopathic Medical Education, formal training is available at only six accredited schools in North America. (There were eight before COVID-19, but two have since closed.) Red flag!

To enter an ND school, a bachelor's degree is required. An average GPA of 3.2 is reportedly desired for admission, but I'm unsure why, as there's no entrance exam comparable to the MCAT for MDs or the GRE for DOs.

Naturopathic school lasts four years, during which naturopath candidates claim to receive "the same" sciences as allopaths, along with holistic and naturopathic approaches to disease. Yeah, right! Examining one program's curriculum, they advertise that the second year is dedicated to learning the medical science of various body systems (neurology, musculoskeletal, etc.), but nearly all faculty members are naturopaths too.

Some naturopaths pursue residencies after graduation, but the ACGME does not accredit them as it does physician residencies, nor are they recognized by as members of the ABMS or the AOA.

These naturopathic "physicians" (and I use the term with great trepidation in my mind) can take the Naturopathic Physicians Licensing Examination. They may begin practicing unsupervised as soon as they pass it, but only in states where naturopathy is legal.

The American Association of Naturopathic Physicians reports that twenty-three states regulate their practice. Some risk calling themselves naturopathic medical doctors (NMDs), cleverly marketing the MD component of the abbreviation, while you are now aware that none of them are actual MDs.

It frustrates me that, although naturopathic services are usually not covered by federal Medicare, they are covered in a few states by Medicaid—for example, in Oregon, where welfare recipients may be assigned an ND (or even a PA or NP) as their "PCP." I feel bad for patients there because I believe they are victims of the exploitation of a population noted for its low health literacy.

In some states, naturopaths can practice without completing formal training. Some establish themselves by working alongside another naturopath or by taking courses online or through the mail. Nevertheless, they assert that they are sufficiently educated to prescribe even opiates.

How come? Because they can.

NDs (improperly, in my opinion) promote themselves as "primary care providers" without having attended MD or DO school, which is why they cannot prescribe medications or perform surgeries in so many states.

EBM seldom aligns with ND's ideology, diagnostics, and treatment methods; in fact, it is likely to oppose them.

Many naturopaths hold dangerous anti-vaccine views (remember that most of the sickest with measles were unvaccinated); others administer ozone intravenously with ultraviolet radiation to "kill viruses and bacteria, treat diabetes, and help ulcers heal." Ozone therapy can lead to severe and permanent lung damage, nettle-like rashes, nausea and vomiting, embolisms, heart attacks, blindness, and more. The FDA prohibits its use in medicine. Physicians who choose to prescribe intravenous ozone may quickly face malpractice judgments and potential sanctions against their license.

For psychological disorders, NDs claim to be helpful. However, I found the following in the medical literature: "the risks to any ill patient seeking care from the average naturopathic practitioner would far outweigh any possible benefit" and "no naturopathic treatment has been clinically proven to be safe and effective for bipolar disorder or any other conditions."

Naturopathy is likely ineffective, harmful, and dangerous. NDs may delay the use of EBM by MDs or DOs, and its practitioners are frequently denounced as charlatans or quacks.

Medical societies oppose the practice and licensing of NDs altogether, believing that they may provide care beyond their educational background and expertise, which could lead to inappropriate treatment of sick patients.

My take is: think twice before spending a single penny on services offered by NDs (let alone NMDs—since that is a contrived title that implies fraudulent practices) because they lack the medical education to provide appropriate care.

In addition to wasting money, delays in making accurate diagnoses and writing potentially lifesaving prescriptions can lead to tragedy.

Don't let frustration over a failure—caused by conventional medicine—turn you or your loved ones into a believer in a more flawed form of healthcare. We allopaths understand you, but we do not trust naturopathy. We view it as an unworthy risk, not merely a waste of money and time.

My dad used to say that in the USA, people have the right to choose how to commit suicide; therefore, naturopathy, quackery, cigarettes, motorcycles, and recreational drugs sell so well.

Avoid placing your trust and faith in alternatives like this.

References and Recommended Reading

1. Definition of Naturopathic Medicine. "*Naturopathic Physician: Natural Medicine. Real Solutions,*" http://naturopathic.org/content.asp?contentid=59
2. Arnold S. Relman, "Licensure of Naturopathic Physicians," Quackwatch, January 17, 2002, http://www.quackwatch.org/01QuackeryRelatedTopics/Naturopathy/relman3.html
3. Naturopaths, "Naturopathic Education," http://www.no-naturopaths.org/naturopathic-education.html.
4. "Code of Federal Regulations Title 21, Sec.801.415, Maximum Acceptable Level of Ozone," US Food and Drug Administration, accessed on July 18, 2022.
5. "Focus: Medical Care from Your Primary Care Provider," CareOregon, https://careoregon.org/docs/default-source/members/education-handouts/pcp-care/hso-physical-health-explainer-english.pdf?sfvrsn+305df314_3, a handout from a Medicaid servicer.
6. "Health Literacy Fact Sheets," Center for Health Care Strategies, https://www.chcs.org/resource/health-literacy-fact-sheets/.
7. https://www.chcs.org/page/WhyChooseND.
8. Willem R. Vroom, "Naturopath Prescribing: The Hill to Die On," *BCMJ*, vol. 51, No. 3, April 2009, p. 101, https://bcmj.org/editorials/naturopath-prescribing-hill-die.

Who Is a Chiropractor, a "Doctor" of Chiropractic (DC)?

A chiropractor (DC) provides chiropractic services, obviously. Chiropractic is yet another form of CAIH.

Chiropractic is founded on the principle that misaligned spines are associated with decreased health, including a diminished resistance to disease resulting from interference with nervous and, consequently, immune system functions. It highlights the body's inherent ability to heal itself, primarily with help from manual therapy, which often involves spinal manipulation aimed at realignment. Some shoe insole stores exploit this questionable concept in their television advertisements. Have you seen them?

DCs view themselves as "primary care providers" with a self-proclaimed ability to diagnose and treat medical conditions. However, chiropractors are neither MDs nor DOs and do not qualify as medical doctors.

Many DCs try to mislead people (check their websites) into believing that their education resembles that of medical schools training MDs and DOs, enabling them to treat sick individuals with equal competence when, in fact, that is not the case.

The history of chiropractic is curious and almost comical, if not for its public health and personal consequences. It began in 1895 with a Canadian faith healer, D. D. Palmer, a practitioner of "magnetic therapy" who claimed to have received the spirit of one Dr. Jim Atkinson, who had died five decades earlier. To that, add the "tale" that he greeted a deaf man at a local bar by punching him on the back, resulting in the man regaining his hearing—if that is true, D. D. must have dislodged some gruesome earwax plugs or reconnected some small bones in the middle ear. Palmer moved to Davenport, Iowa, at the age of twenty and started fixing "subluxations," which he blamed for 95 percent of all diseases.

D. D. Palmer viewed chiropractic as a religion, positioning himself as the "fountainhead" and comparing himself to Christ, Muhammad, Joseph Smith, and other prominent religious figures.

A local newspaper of the time referred to Palmer as a quack who claimed, "He can cure the sick and crippled with his magnetic hands." D. D. Palmer, who called himself a "doctor," was eventually convicted of practicing medicine without a license, which resulted in his imprisonment. He died of typhoid fever, for which no effective subluxation adjustment exists.

Palmer's sons recognized that there was money to be made by punching people on the back to "adjust" "stuck" vertebrae. They established themselves as chiropractors and set up a school for "adjusters" of "subluxations," where a specific number of pounds of force per square inch (psi) punches were taught. And the rest is history.

Chiropractic, far from being discarded, is now a licensed healthcare profession. Today, chiropractors interview patients, gather their history, conduct examinations, perform certain laboratory tests, and create working diagnoses and treatment plans to start, monitor, and evaluate progress.

Why? Lobbyism.

The AMA calls chiropractic an "unscientific cult whose practitioners lack the necessary training and background to diagnose and treat human disease," and therefore, it may be dangerous. It is majorly unsubstantiated by EBM, a fundamental pillar of good medicine.

It doesn't help the profession's reputation when DCs incorporate a variety of unproven therapies into their business, such as colonics, quartz and light therapy, naturopathy, retail kinesiology straps and tapes, shoe inserts, braces, and other gadgets that ostensibly assist spinal adjustments.

Strangely and suspiciously, a disproportionate number of potential clients seem to experience spinal deviations. Right? Think about giving it a try. Or not.

DCs parasitically collaborate with personal injury lawyers resembling the "shysters" featured in TV ads targeting individuals harmed by a "company eighteen-wheeler"—the ones with the deepest pockets. Surely, I don't need to explain the reason, but here's a hint in case you've been asleep at the wheel: $$$.

Despite its questionable beginnings and foundation, along with numerous studies showing that bed rest or massage produce similar results, chiropractic remains popular as a form of sick care, particularly for back pain-related issues.

Why is that? I'm not certain, but marketing appears to be a likely answer.

Chiropractors once treated about 10 percent of the US population, 11 percent of whom were children and adolescents.

To become a chiropractor, a candidate must have ninety undergraduate credits in any subject, and a bachelor's degree is not required.

Pre-chiropractic education has evolved, and it may now require a GPA between 2.0 and 3.5 (which translates to a C to B+ average, not around 4.0 like MDs or DOs); this number varies from school to school, with the average reportedly hovering around 3.0. No school admission test, such as the MCAT, is required. Perhaps more eyebrow-raising, several chiropractic "schools" boast 100 percent or near-100 percent admission rates.

The DC degree usually takes four years to complete, and it is not offered at the same medical schools that train MDs or DOs.

Schooling comprises basic sciences, anatomy, physiology, and neurology courses. Based on the coursework I've reviewed, these subjects are taught at either an advanced high school or introductory college level. Students also receive supervised clinical experience to develop skills in adjustment techniques, spinal assessments, and manipulation.

To practice, DCs must pass the National Board of Chiropractic Examiners test and obtain a state license.

Some chiropractors go on to specialize in fields like sports injuries, pediatrics, or orthopedics. This specialization is designed and conducted by other chiropractors, not by MDs or DOs. But, then again, it is not at a medical degree.

The US Department of Education (now defunct) recognizes fewer than twenty institutions that award doctorates in chiropractic (DC), which are approved by the Council on Chiropractic Education.

The services that DCs can provide vary by state. Health insurers may partially, if not fully, cover some of these services.

DCs may counsel clients about nutrition, exercise, stress management, and lifestyle changes and suggest over-the-counter (OTC) drugs like anti-inflammatories such as ibuprofen and food supplements, despite their questionable education to provide medical counseling. DCs may even order bloodwork and imaging (including X-rays), which they may be ill-equipped to interpret. The X-rays used in chiropractic are often not those that physicians or radiologists would request to arrive at accurate diagnoses beyond scoliosis.

DCs cannot perform surgeries or prescribe FDA-approved medications. Again, this is because to do that, they would need to attend a proper medical school.

Chiropractic primarily encroaches upon the medical fields of neurology, radiology, and physiatry, all of which require graduation from medical school and are recognized specialties by the ABMS and the AOA. It also extends into orthopedics, rheumatology, and neurosurgery (which, as mentioned in previous chapters, requires twelve to fourteen years).

The potential for chiropractic to inflict significant harm is real and should not be dismissed. Well-known and published risks include pain, irreversibly damaged joints, worsened quality of life, vertebrae and other bone fractures, strokes, nerve and spinal cord injuries, muscle paralysis, and delayed proper medical care.

The publisher of an early version of this book told me that she had to stop a DC from adjusting her neck, which a neurosurgeon had recently fused. The chiropractor hadn't even inquired about it. "I went to him because I had not yet read this guide," she said, embarrassed. What a mess that could have been.

I wonder if this DC profession would survive if its practitioners were not "in bed" with personal injury attorneys.

Given the availability of options better supported by evidence-based medicine, such as physiatry, orthopedics, neurosurgery, rheumatology, and even physical therapy, alongside its reported risks, I cannot recommend chiropractic to anyone.

References and Recommended Reading

1. "Chiropractic: In Depth," National Center for Complementary and Integrative Health, US Department of Health and Human Services, accessed on December 14, 2022, https://www.nccih.nih.gov/health/chiropractic-in-depth.
2. Reed B. Phillips, "Chiropractic in the United States: Brief History," accessed on December 14, 2022, https://quackwatch.org/chiropractic/rb/ahcpr/1-2/.
3. Sharon Kirkey and Brice Hall, "The First Chiropractor Was a Canadian Who Claimed He Received a Message from a Ghost," *National Post*, July 2, 2019, https://nationalpost.com/health/the-first-chiropractor-was-a-canadian-who-claimed-he-received-a-message-from-a-ghost.
4. Jeremy Jones, Catherine Jones, and Kenneth Nugent, "Vertebral Artery Dissection after a Chiropractor Neck Manipulation," *Proceedings* (Baylor University Medical Center), 2015;28:88–90.
5. Crystal Conde, "Medicine Under Attack: TMA Defends Patients' Safety, Physicians' Authority," *Texas Medicine*, http://www.texmed.org/Template.aspx?id=20796&terms=tms%20under%20attack
6. Paul Ingraham, "The Dubious Science of Kinesiology Tape," PainScience.com, May 24, 2021, https://www.painscience.com/articles/kinesio-taping.php.

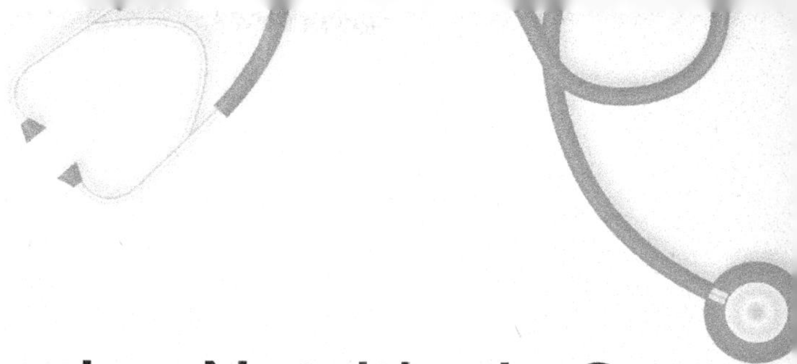

Who Is a Nutritionist? A Registered Dietitian (RD)?

Nutritionists advise people on what to eat and not to eat, explaining how a person's diet impacts health and illness. They analyze diets, recommend meal plans, and educate the individuals or groups they counsel about the benefits and negative effects of certain foods on health and disease.

In most states, anyone can call themselves a "nutritionist." The profession is not federally regulated, so nutritionists are not held to professional standards. This explains why so many appear on TV, radio, print media, and the web, endorsing diets, pills, and more. Many lack formal training in health, disease, or food, which surprises me. (As does common sense.)

A certificate (not a license) to be a' nutritionist" can be obtained in approximately twelve weeks. Even this certificate is unnecessary; it serves as a (sham?) ‘ credential" to deceive potential consumers. There is no licensing for nutritionists.

Some people use the terms "nutritionist" and "dietitian" interchangeably. I say this is incorrect because registered dietitians (RDs) are regulated professionals who require state licensing and credentialing, which adds respectability and credibility.

To become a registered dietitian (RD), a candidate must earn a bachelor's degree in dietetics, nutrition, or nutritional sciences, complete a dietetics internship, and pass a national exam administered by the Commission on Dietetic Registration.

The RD licensure ensures competency through mandatory continuing education programs to maintain this status. This is important because the field is constantly evolving. For example, consuming eggs was once frowned upon due to their perceived link to high cholesterol. This notion has changed, and eating eggs is now considered healthy. Additionally, who knows what legislation may influence decisions regarding our diets? It seems there will be no petroleum-derived dyes in our children's school meals. Is that not bad? It is viewed as it is in Europe.

RDs are not MDs or DOs, and most do not pretend to be. Instead, they collaborate appropriately with medical doctors to provide holistic patient care for individuals affected by diabetes, obesity, renal and gastrointestinal illnesses, cancer, and other diseases.

RDs design and often prepare diets for hospitalized patients, as well as cafeteria meals for their relatives and ancillary personnel, including nurses and doctors.

Neither the ABMS nor the AOA recognizes boards in clinical nutrition. However, a few MDs and DOs pursue credentialing through the American Board of Physician Nutrition Specialists, which they can obtain if certified in certain specialties and able to document 1000 hours or six months of formally mentored clinical nutrition education, including experience in both outpatient and inpatient settings.

MDs or DOs who specialize in critical care medicine, endocrinology- particularly diabetology and obesity or bariatrics (though that definition is evolving), cardiology, nephrology, or gastroenterology may be eligible for fellowships in clinical nutrition.

Advising on nutritional care can be time-consuming, and time is something many MDs and DOs lack. Furthermore, most MDs and DOs would acknowledge that their education in nutrition is generally cursory. While physicians are trained to recognize signs and symptoms of deficiencies and understand basic fundamentals of nutrition, they typically should not, and do not, claim expertise in this area. Consequently, they may not have the capability to address specific issues such as gluten intolerance or foods that cause gut inflammation or ulcers competently; therefore, they refer weight management issues or disease-related nutritional consultations to RDs.

Patients and their relatives should ask their MDs or DOs whom to approach for guidance on diet and nutrition.

References and Recommended Reading

1. "Naturopathy," Wikipedia, https://en.wikipedia.org/wiki/Naturopathy.
2. "Occupational Outlook Handbook: Dietitians and Nutritionists," Bureau of Labor Statistics, US Department of Labor, http://www.bls.gov/ooh/healthcare/dietitians-and-nutritionists.htm.
3. Kari Hartel, "What's the Difference between a Dietitian and a Nutritionist?" FitDay, http://www.fitday.com/fitness-articles/nutrition/whats-the-difference-between-a-dietitian-and-a-nutritionist.html#b.
4. "Where to Get Professional Nutrition Advice, Quackwatch, http://wwwquackwatch.com/04ConsumerEducation/nutritional.html.

Who Should Be Your Doctor?

This chapter is replete with my personal views and biases about the status of health and sick care in the United States.

I will try to avoid sounding partisan or considering economic implications, giving purely optimal suggestions as I perceive them. The goal is to help patients find the best "doctor" for their ailment.

I must repeat the disclaimer that the book is not intended to diagnose or treat any disease or patient; it merely guides readers to the right physicians for themselves and their loved ones.

Some of my opinions go against what public policy, insurers, and even other doctors (and patients) recommend, recognizing that we work within a faulty and progressively socialized system—one that started decades before the creation of the (Un)Affordable Care Act, which tolerates and pays quacks. (The (Un) is mine.)

When the cat's away, the mice will play.

I don't solely blame the government for its shortcomings in management and regulation; I also hold doctors and patients accountable for not protesting loudly enough.

The private sector plays a significant role, which includes medical insurers, certain physicians, private equity firms that acquire medical practices, clinics, hospitals, the legal system, a few pharmaceutical manufacturers, intermediaries, and marketers, including pharmacies.

Lawyers and the malpractice system they exploit, politicians and lobbying (a legal form of corruption), technology that imposes time-wasting, frustrating electronic health records (ask patients), the cost of modernizing equipment, and other factors wreak havoc on the profession.

As much as I dislike overregulation, certain practices-particularly those taken over by private equity firms that hire mid-level providers instead of actual doctors, deserve meticulous monitoring, partly because that system of economics and administration resembles Ponzi schemes. It may be my impression, but you can ask around.

When it comes to the quality of medical care, I prefer subspecialists over generalists. This may sound counterintuitive, but generalists often bite more than they can chew. I previously mentioned my tendency to go against the grain of current healthcare dogma. This philosophy antagonizes insurance carriers and socialized governmental medicine: cost minimization (to them, not to you) at the expense of patients and doctors. We have become so accustomed to this healthcare system that we consider its flawed approach acceptable—until a dear relative needs a second mammogram in a year, and it doesn't get approved.

From a financial perspective, I cannot fault insurers in a capitalistic society. They run a business and must prioritize their shareholders (you might be one if you invest in it on Wall Street) while addressing patients' needs only secondarily.

But trust me, from the perspectives of medical doctors and patients, government insurers do a disastrous job. Not that I claim to know better how to run Medicare or Medicaid, but my excuse is that I am just a physician—it's not my job.

Administrative failures are illustrated by the fact that at the time of billing, neither the providers nor the patients can determine the appropriate code and the corresponding charge due to the complexity and multitude of variables involved. Consequently, patients receive adjustments in the mail or are notified during their next visit. Has that not happened to you? Furthermore, patients often lack clarity about their financial responsibility concerning their bills; thus, many letters labeled as explanations of benefits circulate back and forth, which is why temporary solutions like "surprise billing initiatives" are proposed.

When it comes to government-run, insurance-like programs, it's clear that they struggle to operate practices cost-effectively, wouldn't you agree? The scandals surrounding the performance of the Veterans Administration system and the ongoing need for its revamping serve as notable examples.

Still, patients can count on rights!

Patients have the right to know about the protections and rights provided by the federal government, as well as by state, regional, or institutional authorities. It is essential to familiarize yourself with these rights and understand how to assert them when necessary. A common feature of the "Patient Bill of Rights" is the option to request being seen by an MD or DO instead of a midlevel provider.

I support, if not propose, the following and more tidbits to optimize your medical care. Keep in mind that this is just an opinion, one that is not monetarily or politically based:

1. Remove CAIH providers from your care options. Neither the private sector nor any government agency should cover those services; many advanced countries do not offer them, yet patients there still manage to

thrive. This means you should steer clear of homeopaths, chiropractors, naturopaths, herbalists, snake oil vendors, Rolfers, Reiki practitioners, colonic cleansers, chelation therapists, cupping practitioners, iridologists, or reflexologists, among others.

As with anything, exceptions may occur occasionally. For instance, an orthopedic surgeon might refer a patient to a chiropractor if neither a physiatrist nor a physical therapist is available within a reasonable distance.

2. Seek a specialist (or, even better, a subspecialist) for your ailment as soon as possible. In other words, bypass the generalist if you have a clear idea of what is wrong. For instance, consult a nephrologist or cardiologist for high blood pressure (hypertension); if they refer you to an internist, that should work (they are like orchestra directors), even if it may seem like a step back.
3. Generalists, such as family physicians, are valuable when:
   (a) One needs greater knowledge about a symptom or finding—or some form of triage.
   (b) A preferred specialist or subspecialist is not available within a reasonable time and distance.
   (c) All you need is preventive medicine (e.g., vaccines and check-ups).
   (d) You seek convenient care, such as school physicals and one-time refills while traveling.
   (e) Not much more (in this paradigm).

I believe that generalists divide their time among pediatrics, adult care (including some OB/GYN and family planning), immunizations, various forms of preventive medicine, mental health issues (for instance, refills), minor surgery, and more. Expertise in all these areas becomes limited, diluted, basic, and wanes over time. It is just too many things to keep up with.

One of my family practice (FP) rotating residents described her trade as "one-stop healthcare shopping." A competent and caring FP would be skilled at directing and referring patients to the right specialist or subspecialist.

4. For adults, internists (specialists in internal medicine) are more skilled diagnosticians and therapists (compared to FPs) but are still viewed as generalists by insurance companies.

   Do you know the difference between internists and interns? Interns are in their first year of postgraduate training after graduating from medical school, whereas an internist has completed three years of internal medicine (IM) residency.

5. For women, it may be beneficial to have an OB/GYN, ideally one with whom they have a long-term relationship, for gynecological and breast cancer screenings as well as primary care. However, it may be more suitable for women to choose an internist as their primary care physician.
6. For children, start with a pediatrician rather than a family physician. Consult a general pediatrician for well-baby care, managing minor infections, monitoring growth charts, administering immunizations and vaccinations, and assessing intellectual development metrics.
7. Seek specialized care promptly for severe or chronic illnesses. Examples of specialists for children and

adolescents include pediatric endocrinologists for metabolic or nutritional issues like failure to thrive and thyroid disease; pediatric gastroenterologists for liver and digestive problems such as malabsorption; pediatric rheumatologists for joint inflammatory diseases, including arthritis and lupus; pediatric cardiologists for heart conditions, such as congenital malformations and murmurs; pediatric pulmonologists for respiratory issues like cystic fibrosis; pediatric allergists for chronic sinus and respiratory issues, including asthma and food allergies; pediatric immunologists for recurring infections such as immunodeficiencies; pediatric dermatologists for persistent skin rashes and conditions affecting hair and nails, including eczema, psoriasis, and birthmarks; and pediatric hematologist/oncologists for blood disorders like sickle cell disease and cancer diagnoses and treatments, including leukemia, retinoblastoma, and kidney tumors.

8. Ensure that a candidate providing you with healthcare is either an MD or DO, preferably certified by a board recognized by the ABMS or the AOA, and not a mid-level practitioner.
9. Check the license of any candidate to become your doctor. You can easily do this by contacting the state board where the doctor has practiced. These boards can provide you with the history of complaints, malpractice involvement, peer reports, impairments, any pending issues, and more. Keep in mind that sometimes superb doctors get sued for reasons beyond their best intentions and competence, such as their willingness to tackle severe conditions that others don't. Seek

recommendations and opinions from MDs or DOs whom you trust and have confidence in their integrity.

10. Check websites that report patient satisfaction with potential or established doctors. Using rating sites is valid, but be cautious, as some can be easily manipulated; practice employees may be asked to repeatedly post excellent reviews, and there are services available to protect against or remove negative reviews. A competent doctor's poor bedside manner may work against them. The performance of receptionists, appointment and billing clerks, medical assistants, and mid-level providers may negatively (or, less likely, positively) affect ratings.
11. If asking nicely fails, insist on seeing an MD or DO instead of a mid-level provider, especially during your first visit and most follow-ups. You can always mention that you won't pay or return.

    In many states, regulations require MDs or DOs to initiate all diagnostic and care plans while supervising them (I see all my patients at every visit, even if for just a few minutes; it is relatively easy). It is important to ensure that the work of NPPs is promptly presented to a supervising MD or DO.

    Stand-alone practices operated by NPPs without supervising physicians are emerging everywhere. I suggest avoiding them. Some MDs or DOs own and claim to manage multiple practices at once; I would also steer clear of those.

12. For serious matters, if you learn that a reputable specialist in the disease that ails you is far away (for example, a

rare cancer for which a great specialist is only available at MD Anderson in Houston, Texas), travel to him, circumstances permitting. They usually know peers in your area who could provide proper care and will surely agree to collaborate with your local MD or DO.

13. If reasonable attempts to fix something still fail, seek doctors who have conducted clinical studies on the concern. These have a keen interest in the subject and extensive experience. Helpful listings may be available at FDA websites, or you can ask your physician.
14. If you have doubts about the accuracy of a diagnosis or the validity of a treatment, consider requesting a consultation at a medical school or university hospital. Experts in proposed diagnoses and treatments can be found online or by phone, and you can also learn how to request an appointment.
15. Consider reaching out to the NIH for rare conditions or those your doctors find perplexing (decent ones typically would inform you without any professional jealousy). Caring and skilled doctors can sense when a patient is unsatisfied, which frustrates them and motivates them to help find an alternative.
16. Suppose one thinks that symptoms and signs are putting one at risk of dying overnight or over the weekend or of dangerously worsening. In that case, one should consider, instead of running to a stand-alone ER or urgent care (UC) facility, often run by NPPs, hanging in there for a day or two and showing up at your doctor's office first thing the next morning. I bet they'll work you in. (This is a delicate matter, so take it carefully.)

17. Chest pain and the possibility of a stroke are exceptions; for these, call 911 immediately for an ambulance to take the patient to a hospital they are familiar with.

    Cold symptoms and most rashes are inappropriate reasons to utilize ER or UC facilities, so avoid going there solely for convenience. Additionally, keep in mind that ERs usually have even higher costs than UCs, which are not inexpensive at all.

18. Always prioritize your health. I insist. Don't try to save money by not seeing the best possible doctor for your ailment or by not traveling to the place providing the best care.

    It is well known that healthcare costs have skyrocketed, while payments to physicians have trended down. However, that is no excuse for neglecting to seek medical care that pertains to your life. Shop around to find the best medical insurance you can afford. Some options may be expensive, and finding a trustworthy broker may require significant effort. Ensure that the plan you choose covers your preferred doctors and medications. And don't say, as one of my patients did, that you couldn't pay for your thyroid, diabetes, or blood pressure pills while recounting a recent trip to Disney.

19. Patients should not go to a doctor because ads convince them or their insurer forces them to. They should go because the doctor seems the most qualified. Most better doctors do not advertise; they count on word-of-mouth from satisfied patients.
20. Your MD or DO knows better than the ones you find in search engines. One may ask about what your doctor

thinks of what you found in one, but you must trust your MD or DO's opinion better.

I must end this section with notes regarding my profession so you don't think we can't criticize ourselves or are unaware of our faults.

Medical doctors are aware they may be at fault for a significant part of what is not good about health care,

We also know that we are not all equal in the way we practice,

And that kindness may need to be taught better in medical school.

Other differences in the quality of medical doctors relate to how they are selected for school: no more dynasties exist (which I find sad because it implies that our sons and daughters do not wish to follow in our footsteps). Panic over wokeism, nepotism, discrimination, and inclusiveness-related moralities, as well as family values, beliefs, traditions, and other factors, interfere with the selection of candidates for graduate and postgraduate residency and fellowship programs.

We recognize that good bedside manners offer significant therapeutic benefits. If we could allocate more time to explaining patients' diagnoses and treatments when we do not meet their expectations, we would do so, resulting in happier patients who are less likely to seek out dishonest practitioners. However, the low compensation for our time and expertise significantly contributes to poor communication, a challenge that doctors still need to advocate against. Our professional societies attempt to address this, but unfortunately, they fall short. Regrettably, the most prominent physician organization, the AMA, has a membership rate of well below 20 percent among MDs and DOs.

Computers and web conferences are replacing professors, and soon AI may also do so, which could be for the better. AI may affect charitable work, honesty, decency, sensitivity, and similar qualities- traits that should have been taught at home. Yet, many patients complain that doctors lack these qualities. To me, the issue stems from poor communication skills and time constraints.

AI may indirectly impact the willingness to remain interested in the medical field, study hard forever, and excel. Some doctors who seemingly completed medical school were never cut out to be in medicine; AI may assist them.

In a free economy, patients would deselect mediocre or bad doctors by choosing not to return to them. The number of patients diagnosed and treated should snowball for the good ones. However, in medical practice, we do not have a truly free economy; instead, we face pricing impositions, government intrusions, lawsuit abuses, various business models, and so on, all colluding against decent physicians.

Very few individuals enter the medical field solely to become extremely wealthy, and such individuals should be filtered out during the admissions process. At the same time, no doctor should struggle to afford attending medical conferences due to a lack of funds.

No one takes on the costs, time commitment, intellectual effort, and stress of becoming an MD or DO with criminal intent. Many other professions allow for this much more easily, and you know which ones they are.

Doctors are responsible for not defending their turf to benefit patients and for allowing midlevels to take over a significant portion of medical care. We permitted hospital conglomerates and private equity firms to encroach on patient care, the former by staffing with skeleton crews (for example), and the latter by effectively destroying private practice. Meanwhile, the government remains inactive.

Errors in planning (and I apologize for blaming the government again) have resulted in a shortage of MDs and DOs, especially in certain specialties, allowing midlevel providers to flourish. Neurosurgery, some time ago (due to malpractice abuse), psychiatry, family practice, and many other fields are now undersupplied. This is partly due to insufficient funding for residency programs.

Now that I have suggested to my readers how to avoid inadequate care, let's find the best possible MD or DO for your health concerns. So far, I hope you feel that I have provided valuable tools to help you do the homework so that we can find competent and likable doctors together. However, I can only assist to a certain extent; patients should lead the way in their proper care.

References and Recommended Reading

1. Elisabeth Rosenthal, *An American Sickness: How Healthcare Became Big Business and How You Can Take It Back* (Penguin Books 2018).
2. Emma Freer, "Coming Up Short—Latest Physician Workforce Report," *Texas Medicine*, May 2024.

How to Find a Great Doctor

Below, I provide examples of common or relevant symptoms (like itchiness or pain), signs (things you can see or touch, such as a lump on the breast), syndromes, and diseases (combinations of signs and symptoms, like allergies or lupus), along with suggestions on the type of doctor to consult for each.

I created this list using a "patient-centered" paradigm that contrasts with the "profit-centered" or "population-centered" approach some healthcare payers propose.

Be aware of overlaps among the different specialties and their skilled doctors (as opposed to quacks), whether they are generalists, specialists, subspecialists, or teams. Furthermore, good doctors do not experience professional jealousy.

Here are examples of everyday situations in which patients may be involved. Often, the information seems obvious and easily accessible. Many were selected from job descriptions on specialty board websites, sometimes complemented by information derived from medical texts and my personal experience.

- For chest discomfort (such as pressure, pain, burning, or ache), heart rhythm disturbances (including palpitations, fluttering, or pounding; fast or irregular pulse), high or low blood pressure, sudden weakness, fatigue, fainting spells, anxiety, sudden arm pain or leg cramps, changes in vision or speech, disturbances in limb mobility, and other acute events, call 911 and request an ambulance with paramedics to take you to an ER immediately, preferably one that is part of a hospital. At the ER, ask for an MD or DO, ideally an emergency medicine specialist, to evaluate you as soon as possible. Do not settle for seemingly adequate care from a charming and persuasive mid medically educated provider.

If symptoms or signs suggest heart or blood vessel issues, assertively request an evaluation by a cardiologist—research has demonstrated that when this is done, survival rates improve.

That is not to say that chest pain or tenderness cannot be due to inflammation of the lining of the esophagus, arthritis affecting the joints (and cartilages) between the ribs and the sternum (chest bone), or even of the muscles between the ribs and not the heart; or shingles. Ask the cardiologist to rule those out or in.

Afterward, with less panic, you can be referred to the appropriate specialist, such as a rheumatologist, neurologist, gastroenterologist, or your regular internist.

Please read and follow the instructions you are handed out at discharge time. Many people don't do this and later regret not following it.

Remember not to misuse UC or ER facilities for minor issues, especially if the concern is contagious.

If you have something like the flu or COVID-19, the sooner you start antivirals, the better they will work. Since MDs or DOs were not accessible during epidemics, pharmacists were allowed to test for and treat these conditions. By misusing ERs or UCs, you may end up spreading infections to medical personnel and patients in the waiting room. Run to those when you fear dying before your regular physician can see you.

You might consider avoiding clinics inside pharmacies where you are unlikely to be seen by an MD or DO and where the NPPs who will attend to you may be shielded from malpractice lawsuits (especially at CVS and Walgreens, due to a deal I find unethical). You could be left hanging if something goes wrong.

Be aware that most settings that offer the convenience of quick or urgent care (UC) and emergency care (ER) are not designed to provide follow-up or other forms of long-term care. They will likely refer patients to their regular doctors or a specialist, as they may lack the time or resources to test, diagnose, and, equally important, monitor patients needing long-term care. Consequently, neither you nor they will have any clear understanding of whether they addressed your needs correctly.

- For excessive thirst and hunger, fatigue, frequent urination, unexplained weight loss or gain, sexual dysfunction such as erectile dysfunction, thin or weak bones that break easily (osteopenia or osteoporosis, referred to as "spontaneous fractures"), swelling in the front of the throat (where the thyroid gland is located), intolerance to heat or cold, changes in the menstrual cycle regarding frequency or amount, hair loss, or excessive growth in unwanted areas, it is important to consult both an endocrinologist and a gynecologist. These may be signs and symptoms of diabetes, ovarian or testicular issues, adrenal gland or pituitary gland tumors, and thyroid disease.

- For weakness, dizziness, paleness, cold hands and feet, easy bruising, bleeding gums, unexplained nosebleeds, anemia, low platelet or white cell counts, large lymph nodes, fevers of unknown origin, and recurrent, difficult-to-eradicate infections, early consultation with a hematologist/oncologist may be warranted. These signs and symptoms can indicate iron and other deficiencies, as well as leukemia, lymphoma, and diseases of the bone marrow, liver, or spleen. Anemia may result from blood loss due to a peptic ulcer; the hematologist can determine that and consult a gastroenterologist and, if necessary, a gastrointestinal surgeon.
- For unusual or persistent female genital bleeding, a lump in a breast or testicle, a suspicious growth present for more than a few weeks (preferably no more than three), blood in the stools (which may appear as red or black streaks), changes in bowel movement habits, localized bone or muscle pain, an enlarged lymph node near the site of a previously diagnosed or excised melanoma or other cancer, or if a tumor is suspected to originate from an internal organ such as the pancreas, lung, bladder, stomach, colon, or rectum, consult a medical oncologist and possibly a surgical oncologist if needed.

  These doctors will directly refer patients to other specialists for surgery, chemotherapy, immunotherapy, and radiotherapy, always prioritizing the patient's benefit without going through a generalist.

- For passing kidney stones in the urine, difficulties managing high blood pressure, fluid retention with edema (water accumulation in areas such as the legs), fever with dark urine, the presence of blood and certain other cells, as well as protein in urine tests or elevated creatinine levels in a blood test, a nephrologist or kidney specialist (not just a urologist, who may have addressed the stone passage) should be consulted. Nephrologists also help prevent kidney damage caused by conditions such as high blood pressure, diabetes, lupus, and infections—even strep throat.

In another example of collaboration, if the nephrologist finds out that blood in the urine is caused by kidney or bladder cancer, he will request the help of the urologist and bring an oncologist on board, as necessary.

- A team comprising radiologists, neurologists, vascular surgeons, and others may be beneficial for pain management, especially if the pain is recent, has lasted over three months, is located in unusual areas—such as the pelvis, lower limbs, or abdomen—or occurs after surgery. However, the surgeon who performed the procedure should be notified first.
- For pain causing limitations in the range of motion of a limb or back (spine), starting after an accident, injury, or stroke from nerve damage, or for difficulties exercising due to age or excess weight, consult a physiatrist, neurologist, rheumatologist, or orthopedic surgeon. They may refer the patient to the appropriate specialist or a physical therapist.
- For an acute headache that persists, relapses, or is accompanied by loss of consciousness, confusion, amnesia, dizziness or vertigo (the sensation that the room or oneself is spinning), nausea, ringing in the ears, fatigue, memory loss, or occurs after head trauma (such as concussions often sustained by football or hockey

players), first visit an ER specialist. If it is a chronic or recurrent issue, see a neurologist, as these may indicate bleeding in the brain or its linings. If this is the cause, a neurosurgeon may be invited to participate in the patient's care.

- For abnormal movements, incoordination, persistent headaches, loss of awareness, color flashes, unusual odors or tastes, memory loss, time distortions, muscle weakness or stiffness, droopy eyelids, numbness, and tingling, consult a neurologist. They may suggest inner ear problems, epilepsy, brain tumors, Parkinson's disease, a form of dementia, metal poisoning, or muscle disease, among other possibilities.
- For difficulty swallowing, nausea, vomiting, diarrhea, constipation, a distended belly, abdominal cramps, greasy, whitish, bloody, or black stools, and yellowing of the white portion of the eyes and skin (jaundice), consult a gastroenterologist, as those suggest hepatitis as well as cancer of the esophagus, stomach, intestines, or liver, gallbladder and its drains, pancreatic disease, malabsorption, or parasitic infections.

  Gastroenterologists may subspecialize and consult liver specialists (hepatologists) or gluten enteropathy experts. If older than forty to fifty, get a colonoscopy with one of them!

- For sprains, strains, muscle pulls, ligament or cartilage injuries, tendonitis, or bursitis- common around the knees, shoulders, hips, and elbows, such as those often experienced by tennis players and baseball pitchers- it is advisable to consult a physiatrist or an orthopedic surgeon, preferably one with experience in sports medicine.

If surgical intervention is necessary, you'll be in the right hands with the orthopedist (does the "Tommy John" pitcher surgery ring a bell?). However, if you prefer a more conservative approach, you will likely be referred to a rheumatologist or a physiatrist.

- For decreased visual acuity, ranging from minor blurriness to blindness, corneal scratches, eye pain (possibly due to glaucoma), double vision, cellulitis (inflamed eyelids and orbital swelling), conjunctivitis (including "red eye," which may indicate COVID-19), itchy eyes stemming from seasonal allergies or bacterial and viral infections (possibly herpes), as well as for retinoid anti-aging creams or gels, or growths or cysts on the eyelid, consult an ophthalmologist first, not an optometrist who refers to themselves as an "eye doctor" or "therapeutic OD."

  Even within ophthalmology, there are subspecialists for the retina, cornea, and eyelids (i.e., oculoplastic surgeons). For experiencing double vision or loss of a visual field, a tumor at the base of the skull can be the cause and requires a referral to a neuro-ophthalmologist, a neurosurgeon, and a neuro-radiologist.

- For growths or other lesions found under the skin of the palms, fingers, wrists, or between the tendons or ligaments of the hands- such as fractured hand bones (common in boxers), deep cuts, crush injuries, carpal tunnel syndrome, or ganglion cysts- consult a hand surgeon from either the plastic or orthopedic fields.

- For shortness of breath (SOB), mainly if accompanied by a progressive, chronic cough, coughing up blood, recurrent pneumonia, bronchitis, adult asthma, chronic obstructive pulmonary disease (COPD), tuberculosis, or lung fungus infections consult a pulmonologist.

  If, for example, the SOB turns out to be due to a cardiac condition causing congestive heart failure (CHF), the pulmonologist will consult a cardiologist or a cardio-thoracic (chest) surgeon, depending on the likely cause (e.g., a weak heart muscle from alcohol abuse or amyloid, COVID, or a defective heart valve).

- If you experience joint pain, swelling, tenderness, stiffness (such as "trigger finger"), redness, and warmth surrounding a joint, lumps or tender nodules within or over a joint, muscle soreness, recurrent tendinitis, low back pain, or pain throughout the spine, fibromyalgia, rheumatoid or psoriatic arthritis, or an autoimmune disease such as systemic lupus, consult a rheumatologist. An orthopedic surgeon may be considered afterward.
- For recurrent or persistent fevers (night sweats/chills) of unknown cause and for infections that fail to respond to antibiotics, particularly in immunosuppressed individuals (e.g., with HIV, transplant recipients, or undergoing chemotherapy) or hospitalized patients, ask for an internist specialized in infectious diseases (ID).

  If that specialist suspects that an infected heart valve is causing the fever, he or she will consult a cardiologist or a cardiac surgeon; if the cause is leukemia or lymphoma, he will consult an oncologist.

- Difficulty conceiving after more than six months, repeated miscarriages, any abnormal periods (e.g., blood clots), irregular, painful, or absent cycles, changes in sex drive, pain during intercourse, diagnosed endometriosis, and pelvic inflammatory disease fall under the expertise of OB/GYNs.
- For pain, a lump or swelling of a testicle or within the sac (scrotum), difficulties with erections or ejaculation (ED), penile lesions (warts) or deformities (Peyronie's disease), fractures of the penis, slow urination, hesitation or urgency, burning or pain while urinating, dark or bloody urine, diagnosed urinary tract and bladder infections, especially if recurrent, or the passage of kidney stones, the physician to consult is the urologist.
- For issues related to alcohol or recreational drug abuse, dependency, addiction, depression, anxiety, attention deficit disorder, auditory or visual hallucinations, obsessive or compulsive behaviors, mood swings, bipolar disorder, or schizophrenia, consulting a psychiatrist is advisable before seeing a psychologist or psychotherapist. If abnormal behavior is caused by a brain tumor, the psychiatrist will refer you to a neurosurgeon.

  Psychiatrists may refer to psychologists if the issue does not require prescriptions. Never start by being treated by one of those "25,000 psychotherapists" promoted on television or radio ads!

- Consult an immunologist and allergist for seasonal itchy eyes, runny nose, sinus congestion (particularly if seasonal), wheezing, hives, lip or lid swellings, reactions to antibiotics, analgesics, and other medicines, diseases caused by the body's failure to fight infections, and control of transplanted organ rejection.

If the latter determines that the wheezing is caused by an obstruction in the airway, he will request the involvement of an otolaryngologist (ENT) or thoracic surgeon as appropriate.

- For itchy skin, burning sensations, rashes, bug bites, mite infestations, blisters, pigmentations, acne, warts, cysts, tumors, moles (particularly if ill-shaped, darkening or multicolored, enlarging, rising, or bleeding easily), hair and nail disorders, or acne, consult a dermatologist. Itchy rashes, like chronic hives (over six weeks), may require teaming up with allergists, but those are few. Identifying the reason for the itch may require time, laboratory tests, trying some medications and consultants.

  To catch melanomas early, have a dermatologist conduct annual skin exams, especially after the age of sixty or earlier if you are at risk (fair skin, a family history of skin pre-cancers or cancers at a younger age, and risky behaviors such as tanning bed use and outdoor activities that cause repeated sunburns).

- For lesions on the feet that seem to extend deeper than the skin or are situated between the bones, tendons, and other structures of the ankles, first consult orthopedic surgeons, particularly one known for specializing in foot and ankle care. Also, do not confuse them with podiatrists.

  Consult dermatologists first for skin lesions on the toes, such as warts, corns, nail fungus, and foot fungus.

They will refer you to podiatrists for appropriate care for conditions like diabetes, preventive care, and very thick toenails.

- For earaches, ear infections, hearing loss, tinnitus (ringing in the ears), dizziness or vertigo (a spinning sensation), allergic or infectious sinusitis, snoring, or sleep disorders like apnea, hoarseness, inflamed tonsils, difficulty swallowing, or acid reflux, consult an otorhinolaryngologist (ENT).
- For bowel incontinence, constipation, hemorrhoids, anal pain, fistulae, fissures, or warts, as well as lower intestinal bleeding (usually bright red) due to polyps, rectal cancer, or diverticulitis, consult a proctologist or colorectal surgeon. If the causes of the first two are neurological (i.e., diabetic neuropathy), a neurologist or endocrinologist may be involved; if inflammatory (i.e., ulcerative colitis), the proctologist will refer to the appropriate specialist, which could be a neurologist or a gastroenterologist, respectively.
- For illnesses thought to be caused by toxins or poisons (e.g., household chemicals, environmental agents, workplace exposure) or drug overdoses, consult an internist (like Dr. House, MD, from the TV series, but nicer), a preventive medicine specialist, or a toxicologist.
- For biopsy or surgical treatment of a lung lesion or any area within the chest, including the esophagus (the tube that carries food from the mouth to the stomach) or the trachea (the windpipe that transports air from the throat to the bronchi, which direct it to the lungs), a collapsed lung, or irritation of the lining of the heart (pericardium) and lungs (pleura), consult a thoracic (chest) surgeon.

- For a blocked heart artery that may need a bypass, a cardiovascular surgeon and an interventional cardiologist (the specialists who place stents) may collaborate as a team.

  A cardiac surgeon may also be the preferred choice to repair a damaged heart valve, correct a malformation, or drain fluid between the heart muscle and its lining, among other procedures.

- For diseases that seem to have a hereditary or genetic cause, which are often detected at birth or shortly thereafter and may affect multiple family members, a geneticist might be the appropriate specialist to consult for either addressing the condition or helping couples at risk of passing on a harmful gene to their children.
- Pediatric surgeons who subspecialize in specific issues may best serve children requiring surgical interventions.
- In the case of diagnosed conditions with surgical indications, surgeons should be chosen by their field of expertise; for example, one should not choose a head and neck surgeon for a foot injury. In the case of visceral cancer, a general surgeon may decide to work with a surgical oncologist. In the case of kidney cancer that has perforated an artery, a urologist may prefer to work with a vascular surgeon.
- If a patient with breast cancer chooses a reconstructive procedure, a surgical oncologist may remove the tumor and lymph nodes if necessary, then a plastic surgeon can do the closures.
- If an OB/GYN finds that uterine cancer has invaded the colon or rectum, he may call a proctologist to participate in the care.

- In urgent cases, the patient may need help to select a consultant and must trust the criteria of the initially caring physician.

This list could go on as people visit the doctor for countless reasons. Each situation should be taken into account individually and adjusted to the patient's medical, economic, social, familial, and other circumstances.

The preceding examples are drawn from sources that describe the most common symptoms, signs, syndromes, and diseases that doctors are likely to be asked to diagnose and treat. As I mentioned earlier, I compiled websites from the boards of each medical field: pediatrics, obstetrics and gynecology, psychiatry, and surgery, along with information from textbooks, medical journals, and additional resources. Then, I incorporated a few criteria of my own, as I have seen a lot over four decades of practice.

I know the list is incomplete, and you may not find yourself on it, but please forgive that. This is only meant to guide patients about what they need and want to do when facing health trouble.

Switching gears, I created the following table to illustrate the difference between my paradigm and the current approach in health care (more precisely, sick care). The current paradigm appears to be more "money-centered" than "patient-centered." My paradigm is the opposite.

In the current schema, patients initially visit a generalist, whether a family practitioner, internist, or pediatrician, who then refers them to a more specialized expert. In my schema, a well-informed patient (like my readers must be by now) likely saves time and money and experiences less stress by going directly to a subspecialist, bypassing one or two unnecessary steps. Only if necessary would a patient be referred to another specialist, subspecialist, or—guess what?—a generalist.

Ultimately, if a patient has a well-established relationship that works and likes his doctor, the opinions of both, taken together, should prevail.

This is a guide to address medical problems that are not satisfactorily resolved while avoiding crooks and quacks.

Current Paradigm →	**Specialties & Subspecialties** ↔	**Author's Paradigm** ←
Family Practitioner		
	Dermatologist	Dermatopathologist Pediatric Dermatologist MOHS Skin Surgeon Cosmetic Dermatologist
Pediatrician		
Internist	Geriatric Medicine	
	Rheumatologist	Pediatric Rheumatologist
	Allergist & Immunologist	Pediatric Allergist & Immunologist
	Cardiologist	Interventional Cardiologist Heart/Valve Interventionist Electrophysiologist Cardiac Imaging Advanced Heart Failure Transplant Cardiologist Pediatric Cardiologist Cardiovascular Surgeon
	Pulmonologist	Interventional Pulmonologist Cystic Fibrosis Specialist Interstitial Lung Disease Obstructive Lung Disease Pulmonary Hypertension Asthma Specialist Pediatric Pulmonologist

	Neurologist	Sleep Medicine Specialist Neurocritical Care Smoking Cessation Specialist Pediatric Neurologist Neurosurgeon Spinal Cord Injury Brain Injury Medicine Epilepsy Neurodevelopmental Disability
	Nephrologist	Pediatric Nephrologist
	Physiatrist	Neuromuscular Medicine Pain Medicine & Rehabilitation Occupational Medicine
	Gastroenterologist	Gastroenterology Surgeon Pediatric Gastroenterologist
	Hematologist & Oncologist	Pediatric Endocrinologist/ Oncologist Oncologic Surgeon
	Endocrinologist, Diabetes & Metabolism	Pediatric Endocrinologist Developmental—Behavior Specialist
General Surgeon		Pediatric Surgeon Trauma Surgeon Orthopedic Surgeon Sports Medicine Hand Surgery (Plastics) Hand Surgery (Orthopedist) Thoracic (Chest) Surgeon Colon—Rectal Surgeon
Radiologist		Pediatric Radiologist Diagnostic Radiology Nuclear Radiologist Interventional Radiology Radiation Oncologist Diagnostic Nuclear & Therapeutic Radiologist
Psychiatrist		Addiction Psychiatrist Forensic Psychiatrist Child & Adolescent Psychiatrist Consult Liaison Psychiatry Psychosomatic Medicine

	Urologist	Pediatric Urologist
	Otorhinolaryngologist (ENT)	ENT Surgeon Neurotologist
OB/GYN		Complex Family Planning Female Pelvic Medicine Female Reconstructive Surgery Gynecologic Oncology Maternal-Fetal Medicine Reproductive Endocrinology & Infertility
	Ophthalmologist	Pediatric Ophthalmology Ophthalmologic Surgery Ophthalmic Pathology Ocular Oncology Neuro-Ophthalmology Glaucoma & Surgery Oculoplastic Surgery Strabismus Refractive Surgery
Anesthesiologiest		Adult Cardiac Anesthesiology
	Pediatric Anesthesia	
	Emergency Physician	Medical Toxicology Medical Physics Undersea & Hyperbaric Medicine
	Geneticist	Biochemical Genetics Molecular Genetics Medical Genetics & Genomics
	Hospitalist	Critical Care—Intensivist Critical Care—Pediatrics Critical Care Surgeon
	Clinical Preventative Medicine	
	Hospice & Palliative Medicine	

By closely examining the above chart, one may notice minor discrepancies in what is written throughout the book. However, this table is a useful tool, but not a dogma. Nevertheless, the fundamentals remain intact: avoid generalists (left column) and seek specialists (middle column) or, if possible, a subspecialist (right column) to assist you unless the subspecialist suggests a specialist or a generalist.

My paradigm would probably save patients' time, aggravation, and money if insurance would allow it.

It makes less sense to visit a family practitioner (FP) for a rash than to see a dermatologist or to visit a pediatrician for a teenager's earache instead of an otolaryngologist (ENT). Consulting an ER physician for chronic back pain or an FP is less logical than meeting with a rheumatologist, neurologist, orthopedist, or neurosurgeon. It is also less reasonable to go to an OB/GYN for recurringly passing kidney stones instead of a nephrologist or urologist.

The above schema differs from how many third-party payors want you to seek medical care, which is under the guise that the generalist-to-specialist and subspecialist path would save money; maybe to them, hence my recommendation.

If you are the one with the itch, ache, or pain, don't just go where an insurance company's penny-pinching administrator or triage nurse tells you to unless they threaten you with non-coverage.

Go where I recommend (the best possible doctor). Advocate for who is best suited for you. And ensure you are not assigned to a mid-medically educated practitioner (MEP). Remember that!

Notice the absence of quacks and crooks in my paradigm. I include no CAIH practitioners in it, nor (dys)functional medicine "doctors," homeopaths, NPPs, psychotherapists, and the like.

To simplify, my choices to take care of you and me are, at least initially:

1. MDs or DOs who are members of boards approved by the ABMS or AOA.
2. Whoever those (in 1) refer you to.
3. No one else.

Be very careful; this country may end up with medicine provided by mid-levels, crooks, or quacks if you aren't or don't raise your voice against it.

Best of luck!

References and Recommended Reading

1. Texas Medical Association. *TMA Joins Fight Against Scope Creep in "Sweeping" Federal Legislation.* https://www.texmed.org/TexasMedicineDetail.aspx?id=60784#:~:text=Organized%20medicine%20is%20banding%20together,of%20Medicare%20and%20Medicaid%20patients.
2. Patient's Bill of Rights. http://www.healthsourceglobal.com/docs/patient%20bill%20of%20rights_merged.pdf.
3. Patient Bill of Rights and Responsibilities. http://www.hopkinsmedicine.org/the_john_hopkins_hospital/_docs/bill_of_rights.pdf
4. "When to See a Cardiologist," University of Utah Health, http://healthcare.utah.edu/cardiovascular/when-to-see-cardiologist.php.
5. Healthgrades. *Endocrine Disorders Symptoms.* http://www.healthgrades.com/conditiond/endocrine-disorders-symptoms
6. American Society of Hematology. *Bleeding disorders.* http://www.hematology.org/Patients?bleeding.aspx
7. American Society of Hematology. *Anemia.* http://www.hematology.org/Patients/Anemia/.

8. American Cancer Society. *Signs and Symptoms of Cancer*. http://www.cancer.org/cancer/cancerbasics/signs-and-symptoms-of-cancer.
9. Dr. Ananya Mandal, "When to See a Nephrologist," NewsMedical.net, http://www.news-medical.net/health/When-to-see-a-Nephrologist.aspx.
10. 5 Reasons to See a Pulmonologist. http://avitahealth.org/uploads/images/Brochures/5%20reasons%20to%see%20a%pulmonologist.pdf.
11. Hospital for Special Surgery. *Ask the Expert: When should you see a Rheumatologist?* http://www.hss.edu/playbook/ask-the-expert-when-should-you-see-a-rheumatologist/#.VsR-MvlrLcs.
12. IDSA. *What is an Infectious Disease Specialist?* http://www.idsociety.org/ID_Specialist/.
13. Everyday Health. *When to call your Gynecologist*. http://www.everydayhealth.com/womens-health/sign-you-need-to-visit-your-gynecologyst.aspx.
14. Dr. Zeitlin, MD. *Why see a urologist?* http://www.drzeitlin.com/about-dr-zeitlin/why -see-a-urologist/.
15. American Psychiatric Association. *Early Warning. Signs of Mental Illness*. http://www.psychiatry.org/mental-health/more-topics/warning-signs-of-mental-illness.
16. University of Utah Health Care. *Should you See a Neurologist?* http://www.healthcare.utah.edu/neurosciences/neurology/neurologist.php.
17. Advocate Illinois Masonic Medical Center. *When to see a gastroenterologist*. http://www.advocatehealth.com/immc/when-to-see-a-gastroenterologist-585.
18. Canadian Ophthalmological Society. *When should you see an ophthalmologist?* http://www.cos-sco.ca/vision-health-information/when-should-you-see-an-ophthalmologist/.
19. Healthline. *Autoimmune disease*. http://www.healthline.com/health/autoimmune-disorders#overview.
20. American College of Allergy, Asthma & Immunology. *When to see an Allergist*. http://acaai.org/allergies/treatment/when-to-see-an-allergist.
21. American Academy of Dermatology. *Diseases and Treatments*. http://www.skincarephysicians.com/skincancernet/whentosee.html.

22. Everyday Health. *Should you see a Dermatologist?* http://www.everydayhealth.com/skin-and-beauty/should-you-see-a-dermatologist.aspx.
23. Cleveland Clinic. *When to see a pain specialist. https://health.clevelandclinic.org/when-to-see-a-pain-specialist/*
24. American Academy of Physical Medicine and Rehabilitation. *Why visit a PM&R physician.* http://www.aapmr.org/patients/aboutpmr/Pages/WhyARehabPhysician.aspx.
25. Intermountain Healthcare. Sports Medicine. Mayo Clinic. *Concussion*.http://www.mayoclinic.org/diseases-conditions/concussion/basics/symptoms/con-20019272
26. American Academy for Surgery of the Hand. *About Hand Surgery. https://www.assh.org/handcare/about*
27. American Academy of Otolaryngology—Head and Neck Surgery. *What is an Otolaryngologist*.http://www.entnet.org/content/what-otolaryngologist.
28. Colon & Rectal Specialists. http://crspecialists.com/?s=medical+conditions.
29. American Board of Medical Specialties. *American Board of Preventive Medicine.* http: www.abms.org/member-boards/contact-an-abms-member-board/american-board-of-preventive-medicine/.
30. Genetics Home Reference. *Genetic Consultation.* http://ghr.nlm.nih.gov/handbook/consult?show=all.
31. National Society of Genetic Counselors. *Your Genetic Health: patient information.* http://nsgc.org/p/cm/ld/fid=144.

Who Is to Blame for Crooks and Quacks?

A politically correct answer could be: "ourselves," MDs, and DOs, but I would add "the public" for tolerating if not promoting them (the crooks and quacks). However, that would be like blaming oneself for falling for fake news. Who hasn't?! I think I did it thrice…today.

So, out of bitterness or naiveness, I came up with a scapegoat: marketers. Remember the introduction? We just went full circle.

As this is the next to the last chapter of such a subjective guide, writing it with little redundancy and plenty of clarity took a lot of time, effort, and care.

I consider crooks and quacks those who, oh so cleverly, peddle opioids to kids, pills to make adults "more of a man, and she'll like it" *wink-wink*, or vegetable capsules and gummies that make old people think clearer, feel better, jog longer and faster, with less joint pain, and so on. I also consider crooks those providers who peddle quackery.

Marketers are the proverbial "influencers" of "idiotensers" mostly. They are paid to convince people to take squishy cubes, colored capsules, powders, juices, and more that would return their energy and strength to where they were in their prime, sometimes using passé actors, models, elderly athletes, and likable politicians (as if there were any, for real) in ridiculous TV ads, saying one will feel lasting benefits starting in minutes or something similar, and they do it regardless of principles. Come on, man! (as an elder president would say).

Beware of ads that tell you that if the eighteen-wheeler of a company (with deep pockets) rear-ends you, you should immediately call a chiropractor (instead of an ER doctor or a trauma surgeon), one with many offices that would coordinate your "care," including the economics of it. Undoubtedly, the chiropractor and connected lawyer are salivating over what may come to them ($$$$).

Commercials suggest skipping the ophthalmologist if you don't see clearly and buying glasses from an owl or the optometrist group a TV ad recommends. Others say that if one must raise the volume of the TV, one may as well skip the ENT and buy hearing aids, which sound better, are prettier, cheaper, and smaller than the ones you could get from an audiologist, as your dad would also enjoy when he hears you say you love him over and over. Is that not clever merchandising?

If not for marketers, who do you think patients would go to, good doctors they would find without help or ones that advertise? I bet many would succumb to the latter. Why? I'll answer my question with another question: What brand of pillow do you first think of when shopping for one? One that bombards us with ads by an annoying guy with a dyed mustache who peers through bathroom mirrors, or one better rated in respectable consumer magazines.

And which competitor to the products for weight loss, hair loss, prostate and penis enlargement, and more do you think of buying when hearing "#1 doctor recommended"? Could that be just one doctor well paid as to be unethical? (In my next book, I'll work on teaching how to pull those "fake news" ads off your minds.)

A caveat results from the ways brands are pushed onto doctors and pharmacists. "Used or recommended by more dermatologists," the ad would say, but why? Could it be because free samples are sent to them to try at home a week before a survey? Trust me, when those samples run out, they are forgotten and replaced with the next proven best product in the EBM literature or any other your spouse brings from the discount mega-store. Or "#1 recommended by pharmacists," who knows the enticement? "Dermatology tested" may mean that only one dermatologist performed some test.

How about medical practitioners who convince women that they need lasers, fillers, Botox, or even vaginoplasties (read about the long-term results) to be more desirable and competitive against other ladies in the neighborhood? Remind them about the "vampire" facial, which uses platelets and gave three women HIV. I wonder how many have gotten hepatitis from beautification procedures involving platelets and other cells pushed in with needles.

Cosmetic and plastic surgeons, dermatologists, even OB/GYNs and dentists who really would like to please may talk clients (who may not need anything) into letting themselves injected with botulinum-like products to give them wrinkle-free (albeit expressionless) foreheads and fillers into the lips to plump them up until they are Donald Duck look-alikes, or surgeries that provide them with pointed-up noses, DDD breasts, and more. I have nothing against those products or procedures when honestly advised.

What have those clients succumbed to? The power of marketing.

Paraphrasing Wilde, "I can resist anything but temptation," to which I add "the second half of a doughnut" (a scientifically proven factoid). Keep in mind that you are fighting big money and power and that the ultimate decision is yours. Be strong and do not succumb to marketers. It is you who will pay for the consequences if something goes awry.

I assure you that many cosmetic patients would not repeat their actions, from tattoos, abdominoplasties, and breast cup changes (up or down) to lip fillers and more. They tell me, not you, because they are embarrassed.

Anytime you see, hear, or read about a miracle pill that "supports" the heart, brain, bones, colon, immunity, and so on, before buying it, check what the FDA says about it, its lawsuits, and its marketing.

Medicine is a beautiful career that generates gratitude from many patients and a decent income. Most who practice it enjoy it.

Good doctors must defend their turf from quacks, crooks, anyone who pretends to usurp it, and other marketers of falsehood. And they must want their patients to be protected and benefit from good medicine.

There should be a federal mandate that distinctly separates MD and DO from other professions that call themselves doctors. Some non-MD or DO should be impeded by law and consequently punished from calling themselves doctors, without specifying what kind of doctor they are. As much as I dislike overregulation, it is imperative to regulate the titles that define physicians (and schools of "medicine") so that they will not be mixed up with terms that quacks and NPPs tend to use.

Summary and Conclusions

Excellent health care—more appropriately named "sick care" (because it includes very little preventive care)—likely the best in the world, can be found in the US (socioeconomic issues notwithstanding), and believe it or not, one way or another, it is accessible to all.

Nobody in this country is refused lifesaving care when critically needed (bar the abortion issue in the hands of politicians and lawyers, not medical doctors). However, sometimes, it seems to be at the end of a too-long rope. Social workers, particularly at publicly funded hospitals, can help most find means for access and coverage.

Patients and caretakers may need to take significant responsibility for their medical care and complain less about systemic cracks.

I don't want to hear another "Sorry for not buying the medicines you prescribed me, but they were expensive, and I had to go on a cruise with my beer-drinking buddies," or "I went to a CAIH or a functional medicine physician who prescribed me cheaper ones; I'm back because they didn't work." Patients need to do their part.

With this guide, I hope you learned how to do some of the needed homework and legwork, including how to avoid succumbing to charlatans' ads, not accepting unsupervised mid-level care, and not getting care from most CAIH providers and quacks.

Follow the necessary steps to be appropriately cared for by the right MD or DO. I provided instructions to unconfuse most.

To finish, much of what follows is intentionally repetitious, sorry. It is intended to hammer into your brain what I recommended and dispel the cockroaches (absurdities) that quacks try to plant in it using half-truths or blatantly lying.

Can you tell me why people reply, "Great question," when they mean, "I don't know," and proceed with a speculative diatribe? Or "exactly" and "precisely" when nothing is. Why do lawyers demand 100 percent of MDs and DOs when the most they can offer is 50 percent wins? (As for each case they litigate, another must lose.) What does "It is what it is" mean?

Before you conclude that I am a cranky, biased, and dogmatic medical dinosaur, read the previous chapters to get why "I say what I say," which is not "it is what it is."

Start by remembering that whenever you see "Dr." preceding a practitioner's name but don't see MD or DO following it, ask assertively about the doctorate. Make sure the answer is "medicine." Be suspicious and careful.

When in doubt, call the American Board of Medical Specialties (ABMS)—not so much the questionable American Board of Physician Specialties—to confirm that your MD is certified by the claimed specialty or subspecialty. Do the same if your provider is a DO; call the American Osteopathic Association (AOA) to confirm that your DO is certified by the claimed specialty or subspecialty.

Check with your state's medical licensing body to see if there is trouble with the physician's license and where their practice is located and has been. These processes are more accessible to perform than most people think and will likely be required only once.

Request, or better yet, demand to be seen by an MD or DO and not by an NPP, be it an NP, PA-C, CRNA, midwife, anesthetist, or anyone not closely supervised by an identifiable medical doctor with an MD or DO suffix.

Find the right subspecialist, or specialist, known to treat the ailment that afflicts you or the person you may be caring for, mainly if the problem is serious or has not been satisfactorily dealt with in a reasonable time.

Second opinions are unlikely to offend and be understood by any good medical doctor.

Meet your potential MD or DO to see if you can trust him and feel comfortable with his style, looks, demeanor, bedside manner, personality, appointment scheduling, and so on. Also, check if you would be well treated by the front office personnel (a significant cause of low ratings when not) and if you can like the rest of the staff.

Ensure you can live with the travel time from home or work, the office location, appearance and cleanliness, the parking convenience, and so on.

Also, figure out how available appointments may be and how flexible the front desk is in accommodating patients into the doctor's schedule and not being forced into a mid-level's schedule.

Most MDs and DOs are well-trained, namely because they have completed all the required schooling and residency and are at least qualified to take the specialty boards, better yet, if they have passed such boards and become board-certified.

Understand that not all medical doctors are equal when practicing; some may have excellent knowledge yet suffer personality issues (e.g., inability to deal with stress, marriage and paternity problems, alcoholism and drug abuse, bankruptcy, etc.), which can affect one no less than any other human being. Some charming ones may turn out to be mediocre.

Professional burnout is common among physicians, particularly in some specialties; don't you help to cause more if you want your doctor not to commit suicide, retire early, or move?

A few initially well-meaning doctors succumb to "get-rich-quick" schemes, become crooks, and fall by the wayside, appearing in TV ads and even becoming CAIH. Fortunately, this is rare. In surveys, patients' liking of their doctor ranges around 95 percent.

Sometimes, personalities clash, and a healthy patient-doctor relationship cannot be established. The sooner you migrate away, the better. Exploratory physician changes may be rewarding, even if they confirm good care from your original doctor. There will usually be plenty of good alternatives.

It is in the US where much of the development in diagnostic tests, technological advances, and therapies are invented for the world to benefit. This explains why so many "important" people, like communist dictators, come here instead of Cuba to be saved from certain death. Ask the deceased Chavez whether he, given the chance, would go there again.

Outstanding doctors, superb clinics, and hospitals abound in this country (bar the occasional nut case or scandal), so don't fall for quacks.

I plan to survive or die satisfied with my treatment, well cared for, at practically any medical facility here.

If this book helps at least one person figure out who is the best doctor for them and how to find it by following the instructions to avoid quacks, crooks, and lesser-quality, mid-educated providers (MEPs), (thus saving money and aggravation), it was worth the time (years) and risks it took me to write it.

To end this lengthy last chapter, I add the following reminder: beware of marketers of medical products, particularly those that say, "FDA cleared (or registered)," as that does not mean "FDA approved." Taking advantage of the public, who are not aware of the difference.

Distrust all ads for medical services and products on TV, radio, and other media. Now that you know what to look for, check them.

Good doctors, hospitals, products, and medical services generally do not need ridiculous ads. Some may justifiably inform people about new products or their benefits and alert them of risks, while others may be meant to scam. Good medical care propagates well by word-of-mouth.

It is in the US where I find the medical doctors and hospitals to go to and take my relatives, friends, patients, and all those whom I love and care about, trust me.

Thank you for reading this book. Please don't get mad at me. I realize I irritated a lot of nerves, but I wrote it with the best intentions.

Having practiced and taught medicine for many decades, I know that even the best medical doctors (I hope to be among them) cannot please everybody. But the profession continues to try. You, please keep doing your part.

—William Abramovits, MD, FAAD.

(Fellow of the American Academy of Dermatology (FAAD) means board-certified in dermatology).

I do not represent my specialty or any organization, only myself.

The opinions are mostly mine.

I welcome constructive disagreements and criticisms to help me improve the next edition.

Acknowledgments

I want to thank **Kimberly "Dawn" Vincent, MD, FAAD**, my beautiful and brainy, dear and fantastic companion, colleague, and critic for the last decade and a half. I won't say more to avoid making her uncomfortable.

I want to especially thank Justine Galambus, MD, one of our brilliant residents, who contributed her significant knowledge and enhanced many chapters.

Thank you Abigail Hoffpauir, BS, BA, for your wonderful contributions.

I would also like to thank Saba Suleman, MD, Aselin Puthenpurail, DO, and all the residents of my postgraduate program for their contributions to this book. I greatly benefited from their opinions, time, and assistance.

I want to thank my fantastic team of researchers, Cristina Martinez, MD, and Alison Tran, MD (a former research fellow and now a resident in our program), for their help in completing this text.

Of course, I also want to thank my sons, Alain and Andy; my grandchildren, Eliana and Leo; my ex, their mom; and their grandmother, Bonnie Jean Bible, who had to miss me many nights and weekends while I was working on this book.

About the Author

William Abramovits, MD, FAAD, is an academic and practicing dermatologist in Dallas, Texas. His career started in Venezuela, where he obtained the certification of Physician & Surgeon in 1972. This was followed by passing the USA equivalency by the Educational Council of Foreign Medical Graduates, which allowed him to enter a postgraduate residency program in internal medicine at the University of Texas Medical School in Houston, Texas, becoming an internist in 1976. He then transferred to the University of California in Los Angeles (UCLA) to complete his residency in dermatology in 1979. He later passed the board certification test given by the American Board of Dermatology, for which he maintains certification.

He returned to Venezuela to practice and teach dermatology. Well-known political circumstances there made him relocate back to the US, first to McAllen in South Texas and in 1990 to Dallas to practice and teach, which he does to date at Baylor University Medical Center (now Baylor Scott & White), the University of Texas Medical School at Dallas, and the dermatology residency program of the University of North Texas College of Osteopathic Medicine.

Dr. Abramovits has over 300 publications in peer-reviewed medical journals and textbooks, including several he authored. He lectures on skin disease nationally and worldwide.